Implant Overdentures:
The Standard of Care for Edentulo

Implant Overdentures: The Standard of Care for Edentulous Patients

Edited by

Jocelyne S. Feine, DDS, MS, HDR
Professor
Faculty of Dentistry
McGill University
Montreal, Canada

Gunnar E. Carlsson, LDS, Odont Dr
Professor Emeritus
Department of Prosthetic Dentistry
Faculty of Odontology
Göteborg University
Göteborg, Sweden

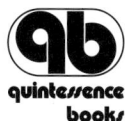

qb quintessence books

Quintessence Publishing Co, Inc

Chicago, Berlin, Tokyo, Copenhagen, London, Paris, Milan, Barcelona, Istanbul, São Paulo, New Delhi, Moscow, Prague, and Warsaw

Library of Congress Cataloging-in-Publication Data

Implant overdentures: The standard of care for edentulous patients /
[edited by] Jocelyne S. Feine, Gunnar E. Carlsson.
       p. ; cm.
Includes bibliographical references and index.
  ISBN 0-86715-430-6 (pbk.)
  1. Implant-supported dentures. 2. Overlay dentures. 3. Complete
dentures. 4. Edentulous mouth. 5. Prosthodontics—Standards.
  [DNLM: 1. Denture, Complete. 2. Mouth, Edentulous. 3. Dental
Prosthesis, Implant-Supported. 4. Denture, Overlay. WU 530 I34 2003]
I. Feine, Jocelyne S. II. Carlsson, Gunnar E., 1930-
  RK667.I45I45 2003
  617.6'92—dc21
                                      2003006220

qb
quintessence
books

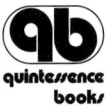

© 2003 Quintessence Publishing Co, Inc

Quintessence Publishing Co, Inc
4350 Chandler Drive
Hanover Park, Illinois 60133
www.quintpub.com

Editor: Arinne Dickson
Production: Susan Robinson
Cover and internal design: Dawn Hartman

Printed in China

Table of Contents

Preface

It is now widely accepted that implant prostheses are a great improvement over conventional dentures. However, most of the evidence in support of this therapy comes from studies of prostheses that require several implants, such as fixed implant-supported prostheses. Unfortunately, millions of edentulous individuals cannot afford fixed prostheses, and therefore most are still wearing conventional dentures.

In the past 8 years, studies have begun to focus on implant therapies that are more accessible to edentulous individuals with low incomes. Two-implant overdentures provide patients with increased satisfaction and quality of life. In addition, these simple implant overdentures have been shown to significantly improve the nutritional state of elderly patients. This information has been published so recently that many clinicians are not familiar with it.

For this reason, we organized a symposium on two-implant overdentures, bringing together a number of expert clinicians and researchers from several countries to discuss their experiences with this treatment modality. In this book, we are delighted to offer the material presented at the symposium, which was held at McGill University in May 2002. Chapters cover topics such as the preferences and treatment expectations of edentulous patients, the benefits of two-implant overdentures as compared with conventional dentures, the predicted costs faced by clinicians in providing this therapy, and treatment planning. The book includes a remarkable chapter in which a classic case is illustrated step-by-step from first examination to recall visits (chapter 13).

This book was written to provide dental students and clinicians with a thorough background to this important topic, so that they can offer evidence-based rehabilitative care to their patients. It will be useful to anyone who treats or who is considering treating edentulous patients.

Based on the evidence presented at the symposium, the speakers and their colleagues produced a consensus statement recommending that two-implant mandibular overdentures should replace mandibular conventional dentures as the standard of care for edentulous patients (see page 155). After reading this book, perhaps you will also agree.

The symposium and subsequent publication of this book would not have been possible without the generous support of Straumann Canada Limited and the tireless efforts of Mrs. Olga Chodan from the Continuing Education Committee of McGill University Faculty of Dentistry. We also greatly appreciate the efficient and expert assistance provided by Quintessence Publishing.

Contributors

Manal A. Awad, BDS, MSc, PhD
Assistant Professor
Departments of Nursing and Health Sciences
  Administration
College of Health Sciences
University of Sharjah
Sharjah, United Arab Emirates

Pierre Boudrias, DMD, MSD
Professor
Department of Restorative Dentistry
University of Montreal
Montreal, Canada

Gunnar E. Carlsson, LDS, Odont Dr,
  Dr Odont hc, FDSRCS
Professor Emeritus
Department of Prosthetic Dentistry
Faculty of Odontology
Göteborg University
Göteborg, Sweden

Antoine Chehade, DDS, MSc, FRCD(C)
Associate Professor
Department of Oral and Maxillofacial Surgery
Faculty of Dentistry
McGill University
Montreal, Canada

Warwick J. Duncan, BDS, MDS,
  FRACDS (Perio)
Senior Lecturer
Department of Oral Rehabilitation
School of Dentistry
University of Otago
Dunedin, New Zealand

Jocelyne S. Feine, DDS, MS, HDR
Professor
Faculty of Dentistry
McGill University
Montreal, Canada

Timothy W. Head, DDS, MSc, FRCD(C)
Director
Department of Oral and Maxillofacial Surgery
Faculty of Dentistry
McGill University
Montreal, Canada

Guido Heydecke, DDS, Dr Med Dent
Assistant Professor
Department of Prosthodontics
School of Dentistry
Albert-Ludwigs University
Freiburg, Germany

James P. Lund, BDS, PhD, Dr Odont hc
Professor and Dean
Faculty of Dentistry
McGill University
Montreal, Canada

Michael I. MacEntee, PhD, FRCD(C)
Professor and Chair
Division of Prosthodontics
Department of Oral Health Sciences
Faculty of Dentistry
University of British Columbia
Vancouver, Canada

Regina Mericske-Stern, Dr Med Dent, PhD
Professor and Chair
Department of Prosthodontics
School of Dental Medicine
University of Bern
Bern, Switzerland

Philippe Mojon, DMD, PhD
Associate Professor in Prosthodontics
Faculty of Dentistry
McGill University
Montreal, Canada

José A. Morais, MD, FRCPC
Assistant Professor
Division of Geriatric Medicine
Nutrition and Food Science Centre
Faculty of Medicine
McGill University
Montreal, Canada

Ignace Naert, DDS, PhD
Professor and Chair
Department of Prosthetic Dentistry
School of Dentistry
Faculty of Medicine
Catholic University of Leuven
Leuven, Belgium

Alan G. T. Payne, BDS, MDent, FCD(SA)
Senior Lecturer
Department of Oral Rehabilitation
School of Dentistry
University of Otago
Dunedin, New Zealand

John R. Penrod, PhD
Health Economist and Assistant Professor
McGill University Health Centre Research Institute
Montreal, Canada

Geert T. Stoker, DDS
Department of Maxillofacial Prosthodontics
  and Special Dental Care
Amphia Teaching Hospital
Breda, The Netherlands

Yoshiaki Takanashi, DDS, PhD
Private Practice in Prosthodontics
Tokyo, Japan

Andrew Tawse-Smith, DDS
Dean and Research Director
Colombian School of Dentistry
Bogota, Colombia

Thomas D. Taylor, DDS, MSD, FACP
Professor and Head
Department of Prosthodontics and Operative
  Dentistry
School of Dental Medicine
University of Connecticut
Farmington, Connecticut

J. Mark Thomason, BDS, PhD, FDSRCS (Ed)
Senior Lecturer in Restorative Dentistry
School of Dental Sciences
University of Newcastle
Newcastle, United Kingdom

W. Murray Thomson, BDS, MComDent, PhD
Associate Professor
Department of Oral Sciences
School of Dentistry
University of Otago
Dunedin, New Zealand

Daniel Wismeijer, DDS, PhD
Department of Maxillofacial Prosthodontics
  and Special Dental Care
Amphia Teaching Hospital
Breda, The Netherlands

It Is Time to Tackle Denture Disability

James P. Lund

Millions of people throughout the world are edentulous. Because they have lost a body part, up to 32 body parts to be exact, edentulous people are physically impaired, according to the World Health Organization (WHO) criteria.[1] Loss of all teeth causes *disability* for most people who wear conventional dentures because they have difficulty performing two of the essential tasks of life, eating and speaking. A smaller number of denture wearers are truly *handicapped* and avoid public speaking and eating with anyone but close family members. These individuals have limited opportunities for success in most professions as a result of the social stigma attached to wearing complete dentures, particularly ill-fitting ones. Denture disability is not a new condition; George Washington serves as a good example. His dentures, which are preserved by the Smithsonian Institution in Washington, DC, were state-of-the-art in the eighteenth century. Dentures like those were available only to the very wealthy. However, they did little to help Mr Washington cope with his tooth loss. He wore them on state occasions for the sake of appearances, but could hardly speak with them in his mouth and he took them out to eat.

There have been enormous improvements in disease prevention and health care since the time of the American Revolution, but this has had little impact on the average denture wearer. The appearance of conventional dentures has improved and springs are no longer needed to keep the maxillary denture in place. However, the mandibular denture is still a horseshoe-shaped structure with no retention and, over the years, it gradually destroys the mucoperiosteum and underlying bone.

The time has come for a pair of twentieth-century acrylic "plates" to join George Washington's teeth and a pair of vulcanite dentures on the museum shelves. Disabled patients deserve better in this new century.

Approximately half of senior Canadians are edentulous (see chapter 1), and almost 40% of them are unable to eat the foods they wish.[2] This means that about 20% of older Canadians could be classified as disabled. Some countries in Europe recognize that something must be done to improve the health of edentulous individuals, and these countries have taken the all-important first step of paying for some types of implant-supported dental prostheses.

However, in North America, much of Europe, and the developing world, edentulous patients are on their own. (See chapter 1 for edentulism rates in various countries.) If patients want implants, they have to pay for them, but most edentulous patients cannot afford the high cost of implant-supported prostheses. Perhaps insurance companies could be persuaded to include implant prostheses in their health care plans, but if the cost of treatment remains very high, this is unlikely. For these reasons, it is very important for researchers and manufacturers to cooperate to develop and test low-cost alternatives to conventional dentures. The mandibular denture is the most critical problem. The authors of the following chapters provide plenty of evidence that mastication, speech, quality of life, and even nutrition improve dramatically if two implants are placed in the anterior mandible to support and stabilize an overdenture.

These chapters provide compelling evidence in support of the consensus statement that was drafted during the 2 days of the symposium on implant overdentures held in May 2002 in Montreal, Quebec, Canada (see appendix). It is time to ensure that edentulous patients worldwide benefit from implant-based denture therapy.

References

1. World Health Organization. International classification of functioning, disability and health: ICF. Geneva: World Health Organization, 2001.
2. Locker D. The burden of oral disorders in a population of older adults. Community Dent Health 1992; 9:109–124.

CHAPTER 1

The World Without Teeth: Demographic Trends

Philippe Mojon

Edentulism, defined as having no teeth, is usually the result of dental caries and periodontal disease. In the case of the latter, the natural course of the disease leads to the loss of all teeth only in a very small percentage of people. The same pattern is probably true with caries, although observational studies are rare. Edentulism cannot be seen, therefore, as the ultimate stage of pathologic processes, but the result of extraction of teeth more or less compromised by diseases. The removal of teeth is related to a series of factors of which the extent of the caries attack or periodontal breakdown may play only a minor role. On many occasions, it is a measure used to prevent future pain, to lower the cost associated with dental treatment, or to avoid anxiety related to dental visits.[1] The number of teeth extracted at the time of full clearance has dropped significantly over the last 20 years in industrialized countries, and today most cases involve the removal of about six teeth.[2,3] Dentists and patients usually agree when full clearance is the most reasonable choice of treatment; however, in 15% of cases, the demand comes from the patient while the dentist would have preferred to keep at least some of the teeth.[2] Among the most frequently cited factors that influence edentulism in a given area are economic wealth, education, the availability and use of professional and preventive services, oral health care systems, third-party payment, dental awareness, and social beliefs. The end result is that edentulism varies widely between countries and also between regions. It also means that edentulism varies over time since the factors themselves evolve over the years.

The gold standard of edentulism evaluation in a given area is to conduct a clinical survey and to identify edentulous people. The survey is the method of choice in less developed countries. The number of people surveyed has to be large enough to be representative and the selection of subjects has to be randomized. An acceptable substitute for clinical observation is simply to ask the question "How many teeth do you have?" The question may be administered in a written questionnaire or by telephone interview; both methods have good validity.[4,5] Hence, it seems relatively simple to

3

measure edentulism in countries by conducting surveys and taking a census on a regular basis. Yet, a review of the data available for the rate of edentulism for the period from 1985 to 2000 revealed that only 37 of the 190 countries in the United Nations had carried out a randomized survey. The information was taken from peer-reviewed papers (11 countries), publicly accessible databases or reports (Canada, United Kingdom, and United States), and the World Health Organization (WHO) website on oral health (23 countries). Information was deemed relevant when the sample was representative of the country and age class (spanning a maximum of 10 years). Only eight countries (Canada, China, Finland, Iceland, Norway, Sweden, United Kingdom, and United States) have detailed data for various age classes and regions.

Age and Edentulism

Despite popular belief, the loss of teeth cannot be considered part of the healthy aging process; however, since caries and periodontal disease are cumulative in essence, the number of edentulous people increases with age. To illustrate this relationship, edentulism in percentage is plotted against age in Fig 1-1. Each of the 286 dots represents the midpoint of a specific age class. When age class was reported as 75+ or 80+, the corresponding values chosen were 80 and 85, respectively. The data summarize 22 countries and 10 regions. Despite the wide spread of dots due to the differences between countries or regions, the influence of age on the edentulism rate is clear. The 65 to 74 age group (value = 70) is heavily represented, since it is a WHO-recommended age group, and so is value 80, which corresponds to the 75+ age group, a common age category in surveys from industrialized countries. A linear regression line

can be fitted to the data to show that, with a 10-year increase in age, edentulism increases by about 4%. However, an exponential model fits the data much better. Both curve-fitting methods are highly significant ($P < .001$). In the exponential model, edentulism increases rapidly only after 70 years of age. One possible explanation is that the last remaining teeth are extracted in one intervention, thus increasing the number of edentulous people more rapidly. This would be in line with reports showing that a significant proportion of teeth are extracted for "prosthodontic" reasons and that the last six remaining teeth are extracted all at once.[2,3]

Edentulism Worldwide

Disparity among countries is wide, as can be extrapolated from Fig 1-1. To illustrate more accurately the difference among countries, the data for edentulism per country for the age group 65 to 74 years is listed in Table 1-1. Criteria for inclusion were that the data must be representative of the country and not a region, and that the edentulism rate must be recorded for the 65 to 74 age group between 1985 and 1999. For example, Canada was not listed because the age classes used in the survey were 65 to 69 and 70 to 98. For these two age groups, the rates were 47% and 58%, respectively. It can be argued that in Nigeria and Kenya, life expectancy is short, and thus the edentulism rate in age class 65 to 74 years is artificially low. However, it is remarkable that not one edentulous person was observed despite the large sample size (4,600 and 1,130, respectively) during the surveys. Iceland has the highest level of edentulism, and this problem has been the subject of several papers.[4] The decline in edentulism is rapid in this country and is being closely monitored. Some similarities between countries are worth mention-

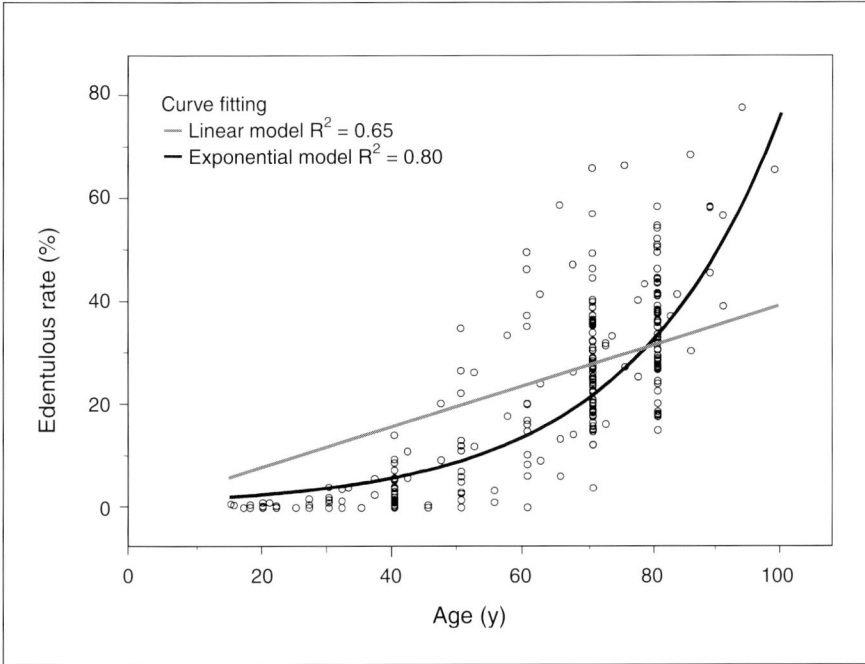

Fig 1-1 Relationship between age and edentulism in selected countries and regions. Countries: Austria, Belarus, Canada, China, Denmark, Egypt, Estonia, Finland, France, Germany, Hong Kong, Hungary, Iceland, Indonesia, Italy, Netherlands, Nigeria, Poland, Sweden, Switzerland, United Kingdom, United States. Regions: British Columbia (Canada), Berlin (Germany), Kitakyushu (Japan), Melbourne (Australia), Navarra (Spain), New England (United States), Ontario (Canada), Quebec (Canada), Rhones-Alps (France), Trondelag (Norway).

ing because they are so different in terms of economic welfare: France and Indonesia have the same rate of edentulism at 16% and the United Kingdom and Sri Lanka both have an edentulism rate of 36% to 37%.

Variation Within a Country

In a US nationwide telephone survey, edentulism was estimated in 46 of 50 states for the 65 to 74 age group from 1995 to 1997.[6] The lowest rate of edentulism was recorded in Hawaii (12%) and the highest in West Virginia (44%), a ratio of 1:3.7. No fewer than 20 states, including New York, Washington, and Connecticut, fall in the 15% to 25% bracket, but for 11 states, the rate was higher than 30%. Such a range could not be found in other countries. In Canada, the Second Health Promotion Survey was conducted by Statistics Canada in 1990 through face-to-face interviews across the country.[7] About 14,000 inhabitants answered the questions related to oral health to show

Table 1-1 Edentulism rate in various countries for the 65 to 74 age group		
Country	Edentulous rate (%)	Year of survey
Kenya	0	1986
Nigeria	0	1991
Gambia	5.6	1995
China	10.5	1995
Hong Kong	12	1991
Cambodia	14.6	1990
Belarus	14.7	1995
Sweden	15	1997
Slovenia	16	1998
France	16.3	1995
Thailand	16.3	1994
Indonesia	16.3	1995
Egypt	17.3	1991
Switzerland	17.6	1988
Singapore	17.7	1996
Denmark	18	1994
Italy	18.8	1993
Pakistan	19.6	1988
Uzbekistan	22.2	1996
Fiji	22.6	1998
United States	22.9	1997
Hungary	27.7	1991
Spain	31	1999
Lebanon	35	1994
Poland	35.5	1991
United Kingdom	36	1998
Sri Lanka	36.9	1994
Estonia	37	1987
Saudi Arabia	38.5	1992
Finland	46	1990
Kyrgyzstan	46	1987
Ireland	48.3	1989
Malaysia	56.6	1990
Netherlands	65.4	1986
Iceland	71.5	1990

that, in the 65+ age group, edentulism varies from 41% in Ontario to 67% in Quebec. In a more recent (1993) and detailed survey in Quebec,[8] edentulism was at 58%, ie, a rate similar to that found in the Atlantic Provinces. The edentulism rate in Quebec remains approximately 1.6 times higher than that found in British Columbia.

Gender Difference

Traditionally, women are considered at higher risk of losing their teeth than are men.[9] However, recent surveys in some countries report a higher rate of edentulism among men.[10,11] To have a clearer view of the present situation, data on the edentulism rate for males and females were extracted from the databank described above. There is a trend for the difference between male and female edentulism rates to increase as edentulism increases, but the variation is wide. For example, in Melbourne (Australia) and in the region of Navarra (Spain), there are 18% and 16% more edentulous females than males in the 65 to 74 age group. On the other end of the scale, in Finland, in the 60 to 64 age group, men are more frequently edentulous by 4%[10] and, in the New England region (United States) at age 85 to 90, this figure is 10%. On average, the female edentulism rate outpaces the male rate by 3% based on worldwide data for all age groups. The difference is statistically significant ($P < .001$) but may not be in the near future. In fact, there is a trend toward the difference disappearing over time. In Finland, edentulism among the working population (15 to 65 years) has been monitored since 1978.[10] Figure 1-2 presents the change over time for men and women separately. In 1997, the edentulous rate for females was lower than that of males for the first time, although not significantly. Similar figures pub-

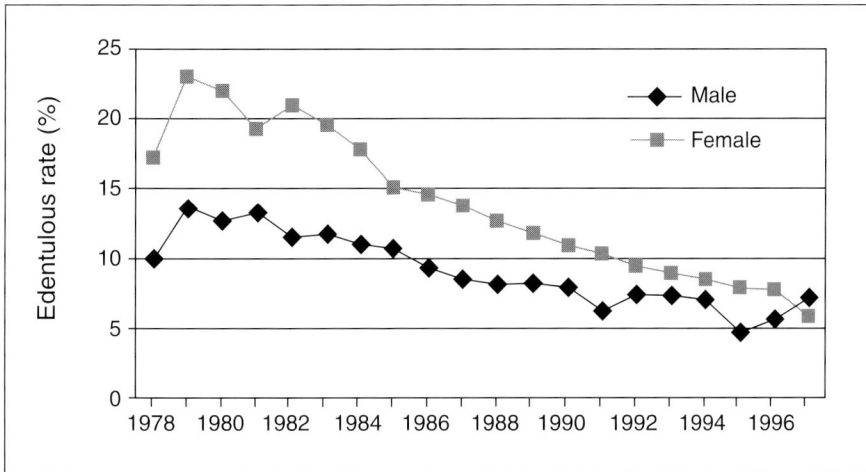

Fig 1-2 The decline in edentulism in Finland by gender. (Data from Suominen-Taipale et al.[10])

lished for the United Kingdom every 10 years show that the rate of edentulism in men decreased from 25% in 1978 to 10% in 1998.[3] However, the difference between genders did not disappear, as was the case in Finland, since the female edentulous rate was still 5% higher than that of the male edentulous rate in 1998. This difference between the two countries may be attributed in part to the sampling of only the active population (15 to 65 year olds) in the Finnish statistics, thus excluding the older age group that was included in the British statistics (age group: 16+ years).

The change observed in Finland has been attributed to women obtaining dental care more frequently and thus having their teeth extracted at an earlier age. With the change in treatment principle and increase in dental awareness, the pattern disappeared.[10] It is therefore likely that the observed difference between men and women is related to behavioral and cultural factors rather than a greater propensity for periodontal disease or caries.

Socioeconomic Factors

Education

Education consistently has been reported as a factor explaining part of the variation in the rate of edentulism.[12,13] It appears that, as a society becomes more educated, it attaches more importance to the preservation of teeth. Based on the data from the Canadian Health Promotion Survey from 1990, the 10% of the population aged 15 to 98 with the least education (elementary school or less) has an edentulous rate of about 50%, while only 4% of those who attended college were edentulous.[7] In the United States, data extracted from the Third National Health and Nutrition Survey (NHANES III) 1988 to 1994 showed a similar pattern: For those with 0 to 8 years of schooling, the edentulous rate was 22%; for 9 to 11 years, 12 years, and more than 12 years of schooling, the rates were 12%, 8%, and 5%, respectively. A few authors[10,14–16] have reported on the relative risk (odds ratio) for edentulism in people with little education versus more education, while controlling other factors such as income and gender. The odds ratios reported are all around 2, ie, the risk of being edentulous is about twice as high among less educated people. However, in Finland[7] this odds ratio was 7.3 in 1978 and decreased to 5.1 in 1997. It appears that, with time, the influence of education on edentulism diminishes.

Income

The extraction of all teeth and their replacement by a denture is frequently the least expensive treatment and is considered (fallaciously) by many as an acceptable means of restoring esthetic function. Therefore it is not surprising to find that income is a strong predictor of edentulism within a country.[12,13] Yet data relating to income rarely is complete, because people are reluctant to answer the question. Nevertheless, the data from the NHANES III survey demonstrates the relationship clearly: United States residents with a household income of less than US $10,000 had an edentulism rate of 18%; whereas for those with a household income of US $10,000 to $29,999; $30,000 to $49,999; and more than $50,000, the edentulism rates were 12%, 6%, and 4%, respectively. The response rate was 58%, and only 2% of non-respondents

were edentulous, suggesting that the non-respondents were mainly among the group with the highest income. Similar results have been reported by others in the United States[14,17] and in Sweden and Denmark.[12,15] Because income is strongly associated with edentulism, mode of payment and dental care systems may encourage people to retain their teeth. In a recent paper, edentulism was compared in Denmark and Sweden, two countries with similar economic and cultural environments.[18] Two samples of residents were matched for age to show that edentulism was almost twice as large in the Danish sample (9.4%) as in the Swedish sample (4.8%), where the government was subsidizing dental treatment. Other studies in different countries will be needed before a definitive conclusion can be drawn on the effect of dental care systems on edentulism; however, current evidence indicates that edentulism can be influenced by societal decisions promoting oral health.

Economic Development

Given that economic factors can explain part of the variation in edentulism within a country, an attempt was made at linking the economic wealth of a country to its edentulous rate. In Fig 1-3, edentulism for the 35 countries with data at age 70 (65 to 74 age group) is plotted against the annual gross domestic product (GDP) per capita for the year 2000.[19] Among the countries with a GDP lower than US $10,000, a regression line is fitted to show that edentulism doubles when the GDP increases from approximately $2,000 to $9,500. The wealthier countries are more scattered and, although the general tendency is for a negative correlation, the scattering of data combined with the small data set precludes any definitive conclusion. From these two tendencies, it is expected that edentulism increases in accor-

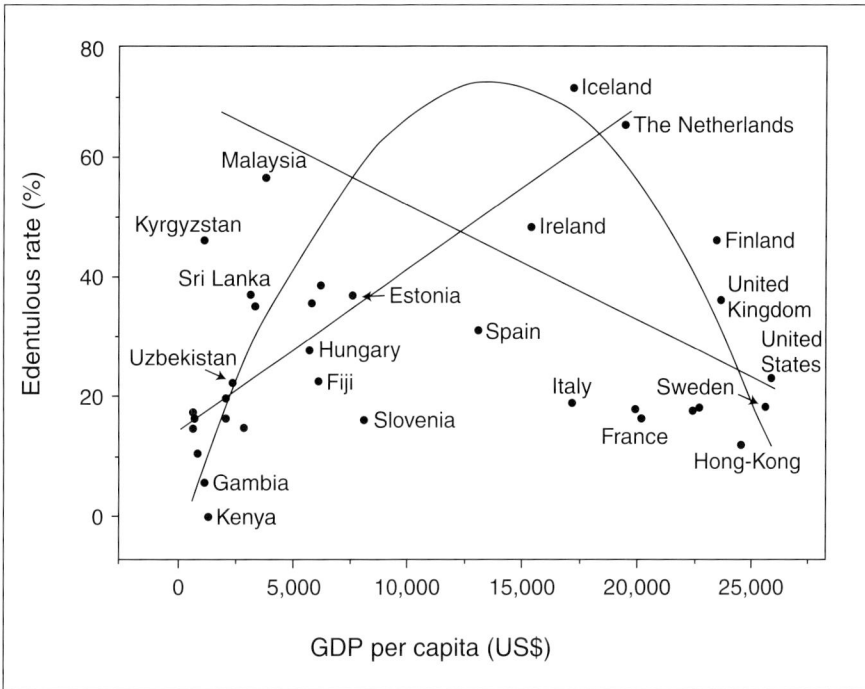

Fig 1-3 Edentulous rate of 70-year-olds and gross domestic products for selected countries in the year 2000.

dance with the wealth of a country, eventually reaches a maximum, and then decreases as the GDP increases. This theoretical model would result in a curve similar to the black bell curve line indicated on the data plot.

Rural Versus Urban

In industrialized countries, edentulism is usually higher in the rural areas than in the cities. For example, in Finland, the rate of edentulism is three times higher in rural areas compared to the capital city area.[20] In the United States, results extracted from the NHANES III survey indicated that the odds of being edentulous in a rural area are about twice as high as they are in urban areas. In a survey conducted in the Netherlands, the number of people becoming edentulous was twice as high in rural areas compared with urban areas.[21] Even when the analysis took into account the level of education and income, the adjusted rate was still higher in rural areas. The difference traditionally is attributed to a lower dentist-patient ratio in rural areas, in addition to cultural factors. In countries where the dental workforce is insufficient, edentulism in cities may exceed the rate found in rural areas. In China, for example, edentulism is at 8% among the 60+ age group in rural areas, compared to 11% in the cities.

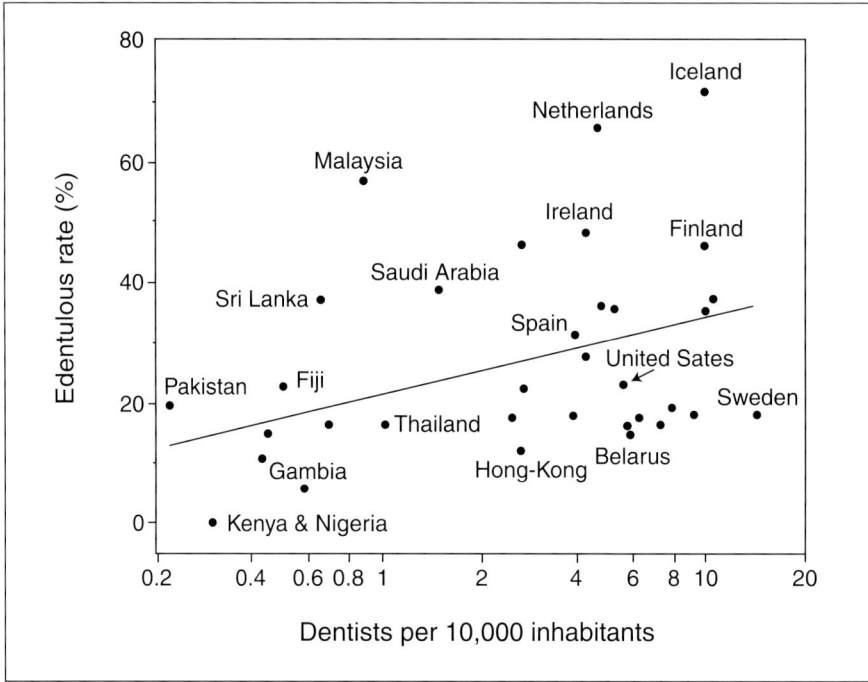

Fig 1-4 Edentulism and the correlation to the dental workforce (dentists and dental therapists) in selected countries. Information on the dental workforce was extracted from the WHO website.[22]

Density of Dentists

If access to treatment influences edentulism, countries with different dentist-patient ratios should have different rates. The relationship is presented in Fig 1-4, where the dentist-patient ratio is plotted against the percent of edentulism around age 70 (65 to 74) for various countries. Dental therapists were included in the dental workforce because they play a major role in several countries. The relationship is not linear and a logarithmic scale is used for the x-axis. The regression line is highly

significant ($P = .01$) and demonstrates that edentulism increases as the dental workforce increases. One would expect that, when the density of dentists reaches a certain level, the edentulism rate would decrease. However, such a phenomenon is not observable in the data presented here. The variation in edentulism among countries with similar high density of dentists is wide (see Table 1-1); for example, Denmark, Finland, and Iceland have almost identical density of dentists. This variation probably conceals the expected drop in edentulism.

Health, Lifestyle, and Psychosocial Factors

It has long been established that oral health is closely related to general health; therefore, edentulism is found more frequently among sick and frail older adults. Institutionalized elderly patients frequently are more edentulous compared to their community-dwelling counterparts,[23] for example. Several reports have shown that smokers are more likely to be edentulous in old age.[13,15] The deleterious effect of smoking on the periodontium makes it a predisposing factor for tooth loss. The magnitude of the effect varies from one study to another, from a mere 6% increase[24] to a 4.5 times higher risk of being edentulous.[25] Cardiovascular disease and diabetes also have been independently associated with edentulism.[26,27] The reason for such associations between systemic diseases and oral health remains unclear; however, it is prudent to view it as a compounding effect due to health behavior or genetically predisposing factors rather than as a true causal relationship.

Psychologic factors certainly are responsible for an individual becoming edentulous. For example, depression has been associated with edentulism.[28] In a study aimed at understanding the reason for full-mouth extractions, dental anxiety emerged as the strongest psychologic characteristic of people who became edentulous.[1] The full impact of these diseases or psychologic conditions on the rate of edentulism remains unknown.

Explaining Edentulism

Several attempts have been made to explain the variation in edentulism observed in different regions of a country or in various subgroups of a population. Gender, education, income, occupation, and age are usually retained in statistical models predicting edentulism; however, it is difficult to find information quantifying variance as explained by these models. In Sweden, a model based on age, education, income, residence, and marital status correctly predicted 93% of those completely edentulous.[12] However, for the United States, a similar model correctly predicted the dental status of only 74% of the cases among middle-aged and older adults.[17] According to the data from the Canadian Health Promotion survey, age, marital status, income, and education were the best predictors of edentulism, but could explain only 46% of the edentulous cases.[7] Age was the primary predictor while the other variables contributed only marginally. Therefore, it appears that, for similar age groups, the known predictors of edentulism, ie, socioeconomic factors and gender, can explain only a small percentage of the observed wide variation in edentulism. Other determinants, such as cultural and dental attitude, must play an important role, but it is difficult to quantify their influence.

Decline in Edentulism

Data on the change in edentulism rate over time exists only for a few countries. Figure 1-2 illustrates the decline in edentulism in Finland,[7] where the decrease was approximately 0.7% per year between 1978 and 1997 for the total population. In Sweden, the rate was also around 1% per year when measured between 1975 and 1996. For the United States, the decline in edentulism seems less rapid: in 1961 the rate was 17%; in 1972, 14.7%; and in 1991, 7.5%.[29,30] These values are evaluated for the whole population. When data are broken down by age, the decrease is more dramatic in the older age group. In Sweden, for example, the decrease is about 0.8% per year for people aged 50 years, compared to 1.8% per year for those aged 75 years.[11] In the United Kingdom, edentulism dropped from 40% in 1968 to 6% in 1998 for the 45 to 54 age group. The corresponding figures for the 65 to 74 age group are 79% in 1968 and 34% in 1998, which translate to yearly declines of 1.1% (45 to 54 age group) and 1.5% (65 to 74 age group). In Quebec, where edentulism is one of the highest in Canada, the decrease rate per year is only slightly lower than in the United Kingdom, at about 0.1% according to two surveys conducted in 1980 and 1993. There seems to be no similar data for less developed countries, and applying the decrease rate taken from the examples above would be highly speculative. In fact, an initial increase of edentulism in these countries as the economy and social welfare improves can be expected (see Fig 1-3).

Projection for the Future: Treatment Needs for Edentulous Arches

It seems doubtful that edentulism will be eradicated in the next 20 years, despite all the effort put into oral disease prevention and treatment. A realistic sustainable goal for the edentulism rate would be approximately 10% for age 70, based on the available data (see Table 1-1). A logarithmic decrease can be expected with, at some point, a slowdown in the decline. Such a model has been used to predict the edentulism rate in the United Kingdom for several age groups for the next 50 years. According to this prediction, the rate of edentulism should be stable at around 3% starting in 2008 for the 45 to 54 age group, while for the oldest age group (75+) the decline will continue until the year 2048. The plateau should be reached in 2028 for the 65 to 74 age group, with the predicted edentulism rate at 10%.

In light of these figures, will there be a substantial need for the provision of complete dentures in the future? In most countries the percentage of aging adults will increase over the next few decades, if not longer. In the United States, by year 2015, the population aged 65+ will increase by 25% compared to the year 1997.[31] In Canada, the latest projection from Statistics Canada predicts an increase of 24% from 2001 to 2011.[32]

The question, therefore, can be re-worded as follows: Will the growth of the older part of the population overtake the logarithmic decline in edentulism?

This question was recently addressed in the United States.[33] The need for complete denture treatment was estimated for the next 20 years based on a formula that took into account demographic projection, proportion of subjects with one or two edentulous arches in 1991, declining trends in edentulism, and utilization rate. The latter was estimated at 90% since about 10% of people do not wear a denture in their edentulous arch. The projection shows a steady increase in the demand for treatment of edentulous arches over the next 20 years. The number of edentulous arches in the United States will increase by approximately 230,000 units every year. The situation in Europe may be more complicated, since the decline in edentulism is more rapid and demographic projections vary markedly from one country to another. Nevertheless, if there is a decline in need for the treatment of edentulous arches, it cannot be as steep as the decline in edentulism.

Conclusion

Since periodontal disease and caries have a cumulative deleterious effect on the dentition, the percentage of edentulous people increases with age. The increase is exponential and rises sharply around 70 years of age. For a specific age group, the disparity between edentulous rates among countries or regions is striking. In the 1990s, the edentulism rate was between 48% and 72% for adults aged 65 to 74 years in countries including Ireland, the Netherlands, and Iceland, while only 15% to 18% of people living in France, Indonesia, Switzerland, Denmark, or Sweden were edentulous. In less developed countries, edentulism is positively correlated to economic wealth. Overall, less educated, poor, and rural patients are more likely to be edentulous, but these socioeconomic determinants only partially explain the disparity between countries or regions. Cultural and psychosocial factors must play an important role as well. Edentulism is declining at a rate of about 1% per year for the total population in most industrialized countries. The decline is more rapid in the oldest age groups. On the other hand, the average life expectancy has risen from 45 to 75 years in industrialized countries over the last century and the number of people aged 65 years or older is increasing in all countries. North American projections show that, in absolute number, the demographic growth will outpace the decline in edentulism. While this scenario may not be applicable to European countries, a rapid decrease of the need for treatment of edentulous arches (using complete dentures, implant overdentures, or implant-supported prostheses) cannot be expected within the next 10 years.

References

1. Bouma J, Uitenbroek D, Westert G, Schaub RM, van de Poel F. Pathways to full mouth extraction. Community Dent Oral Epidemiol 1987;15:301–305.
2. Takala L, Utriainen P, Alanen P. Incidence of edentulousness, reasons for full clearance, and health status of teeth before extractions in rural Finland. Community Dent Oral Epidemiol 1994;22:254–257.
3. Steele JG, Treasure E, Pitts NB, Morris J, Bradnock G. Total tooth loss in the United Kingdom in 1998 and implications for the future. Br Dent J 2000;189:598–603.
4. Axelsson G, Helgadottir S. Edentulousness in Iceland in 1990. A national questionnaire survey. Acta Odontol Scand 1995;53:279–282.
5. Gilbert GH, Duncan RP, Kulley AM. Validity of self-reported tooth counts during a telephone screening interview. J Public Health Dent 1997;57:176–180.
6. Total tooth loss among persons aged > or = 65 years—Selected states, 1995–1997. MMWR Morb Mortal Wkly Rep 1999;48:206–210.
7. Health Promotion Survey Canada, 1990. Statistics Canada. Available at: www.statcan.ca/english/sdds/3828.htm. Accessed April 30, 2003.
8. Brodeur JM, Benigeri M, Naccache H, Olivier M, Payette M. Trends in the level of edentulism in Quebec between 1980 and 1993 [in French]. J Can Dent Assoc 1996;62:159–160,162–166.
9. Budtz-Jorgensen E. Epidemiology. In: Dental and Prosthetic Status of Older Adults. Chicago: Quintessence, 1999:1–21.
10. Suominen-Taipale AL, Alanen P, Helenius H, Nordblad A, Uutela A. Edentulism among Finnish adults of working age, 1978-1997. Community Dent Oral Epidemiol 1999;27:353–365.
11. Osterberg T, Carlsson GE, Sundh V. Trends and prognoses of dental status in the Swedish population: Analysis based on interviews in 1975 to 1997 by Statistics Sweden. Acta Odontol Scand 2000;58:177–182.
12. Palmqvist S, Soderfeldt B, Arnbjerg D. Explanatory models for total edentulousness, presence of removable dentures, and complete dental arches in a Swedish population. Acta Odontol Scand 1992;50:133–139.
13. Eklund SA, Burt BA. Risk factors for total tooth loss in the United States; Longitudinal analysis of national data. J Public Health Dent 1994;54:5–14.
14. Marcus SE, Kaste LM, Brown LJ. Prevalence and demographic correlates of tooth loss among the elderly in the United States. Spec Care Dentist 1994;14:123–127.
15. Osterberg T, Carlsson GE, Sundh W, Fyhrlund A. Prognosis of and factors associated with dental status in the adult Swedish population, 1975-1989. Community Dent Oral Epidemiol 1995;23:232–236.

16. Unell L, Soderfeldt B, Halling A, Birkhed D. Explanatory models for oral health expressed as number of remaining teeth in an adult population. Community Dent Health 1998;15:155–161.

17. Dolan TA, Gilbert GH, Duncan RP, Foerster U. Risk indicators of edentulism, partial tooth loss and prosthetic status among black and white middle-aged and older adults. Community Dent Oral Epidemiol 2001;29:329–340.

18. Palmqvist S, Soderfeldt B, Vigild M. Influence of dental care systems on dental status. A comparison between two countries with different systems but similar living standards. Community Dent Health 2001; 18:16–19.

19. The World Bank data and statistics website. Available at: www.worldbank.org/data/quickreference/ quickref.html. Accessed: May 15, 2002.

20. Tuominen R, Rajala M, Paunio I. The association between edentulousness and the accessibility and availability of dentists. Community Dent Health 1984;1:201–206.

21. Bouma J, van de Poel F, Schaub RM, Uitenbroek D. Differences in total tooth extraction between an urban and a rural area in the Netherlands. Community Dent Oral Epidemiol 1986;14:181–183.

22. WHO Oral Health Country/Area Profile Programme website. Available at: www.whocollab.od.mah.se/ countriesalphab.html. Accessed: April 30, 2003.

23. Slade GD, Locker D, Leake JL, Price SA, Chao I. Differences in oral health status between institutionalized and non-institutionalized older adults. Community Dent Oral Epidemiol 1990;18:272–276.

24. Axelsson P, Paulander J, Lindhe J. Relationship between smoking and dental status in 35-, 50-, 65-, and 75-year-old individuals. J Clin Periodontol 1998;25: 297–305.

25. Krall EA, Dawson-Hughes B, Garvey AJ, Garcia RI. Smoking, smoking cessation, and tooth loss. J Dent Res 1997;76:1653–1659.

26. Hamasha AA, Hand JS, Levy SM. Medical conditions associated with missing teeth and edentulism in the institutionalized elderly. Spec Care Dentist 1998;18: 123–127.

27. Slade GD, Offenbacher S, Beck JD, Heiss G, Pankow JS. Acute-phase inflammatory response to periodontal disease in the US population. J Dent Res 2000;79:49–57.

28. Anttila SS, Knuuttila ML, Sakki TK. Relationship of depressive symptoms to edentulousness, dental health, and dental health behavior. Acta Odontol Scand 2001;59:406–412.

29. Warren JJ, Watkins CA, Cowen HJ, Hand JS, Levy SM, Kuthy RA. Tooth loss in the very old: 13-15-year incidence among elderly Iowans. Community Dent Oral Epidemiol 2002;30:29–37.

30. Marcus SE, Drury TF, Brown LJ, Zion GR. Tooth retention and tooth loss in the permanent dentition of adults: United States, 1988–1991. J Dent Res 1996;75(spec no):684–695.

31. Thompson GW, Kreisel PS. The impact of the demographics of aging and the edentulous condition on dental care services. J Prosthet Dent 1998;79: 56–59.

32. Population projections for Canada, provinces, and territories, 2000–2026 [catalogue no. 91-520-XPB]. Ottawa, Ontario: Statistics Canada, March 13, 2001.

33. Douglass CW, Shih A, Ostry L. Will there be a need for complete dentures in the United States in 2020? J Prosthet Dent 2002;87:5–8.

CHAPTER 2

Edentulism, Digestion, and Nutrition

José A. Morais and J. Mark Thomason

This chapter reviews current evidence of the consequences of tooth loss on dietary patterns and the effect of conventional prosthetic rehabilitation. It also details the effect of implant-supported prostheses on patients' perceived ability to chew as well as changes in patients' posttreatment food selection patterns. The potential effect of these changes on nutritional status is illustrated with pilot data from a study of mandibular overdentures supported by two implants.

Masticatory Process

Eating replaces the body's nutrients, thereby facilitating the maintenance of body composition. Mastication is the first step in this process and prepares the bolus of food for the alimentary tract. Yet the process of eating is more complex than the act of mastication. The process of converting the food into a bolus to be swallowed is associated with the release of molecules from the food that stimulates the olfactory and taste receptors, enhancing enjoyment of the food experience. This process is, however, highly dependent on a functioning dentition, which is an integral part of a healthy mouth, which in turn influences diet and nutrition. The presence of prostheses, or more simply the number and distribution of teeth, influences the ease of chewing and the pleasure derived from different foods. Older adults with fewer teeth than their younger counterparts rely on some form of dental prosthesis to aid mastication. These changes in dentition, in turn, are associated with masticatory efficiency and ability.[1] Nevertheless, patients can and do function well with a less-than-complete dentition. This is the concept of the "shortened dental arch" proposed in the early 1980s[2]: Dental resources preserve a dentition that provides adequate functional arrangement. This concept is a widely adopted treatment strategy.[3] When there are fewer than 21 remaining teeth, however, there is an increasing reliance on removable prostheses,[4] although masticatory efficiency with fewer teeth will be reduced even with a prosthesis.

Although teeth may not be a prerequisite for digestion, at least in the young,[5] a reduced tooth number can make mastication more difficult and lead to the avoidance of specific foods that require rigorous chewing. As the tooth count decreases, patients are more likely to practice forms of food avoidance or dietary restriction. In particular they tend to avoid hard and tough foods that are difficult to chew; this has been well described in patients with oral impairment.[6–8] An impaired dentition in geriatric patients also may render food digestion more complicated, because they may have reduced gastric secretion, intestinal mobility, and changes in absorption patterns. Such changes in food selection patterns can cause patients to favor more highly processed foods at the expense of harder, coarser, and more difficult-to-chew foods. This change in food selection also may lead to a dietary deficiency with regard to vitamins, minerals, fiber, and proteins and may lead to calorific compensation of a diet higher in fats and cholesterol. Indeed, even edentulous health care professionals have been shown to eat fewer vegetables and less dietary fiber than those with 25 teeth or more.[9] Some dietary changes have been directly associated with colon cancer, cardiovascular disease, and stroke. For example, it has been hypothesized that a reduction of 1 g of dietary fiber could result in a 4% increase in the risk of myocardial infarction,[10] and an elevation of 1 mmol/L of homocysteine (associated with low vitamins B_{12}, B_6, and folate) could lead to a 10% increase in cardiovascular disease.[11]

Nutrient Intake and Dentition

Changes in the ability to eat food also are apparent in nutrition intake. Edentulous individuals living independently have been shown to have a lower nutrient intake compared with dentate adults.[12] Those with 21 or more teeth consumed more of most nutrients, especially the nonstarch polysaccharides (dietary fiber), while edentulous adults consumed less nonstarch polysaccharides, protein, calcium, non-

heme iron, niacin, and vitamin C. It also was found that mean daily intake of nutrients and total caloric intake correspondingly increased with the number of teeth.[13] In older patients, a greater number of occluding pairs of teeth was associated with higher consumption of intrinsic and milk sugars in addition to more nonstarch polysaccharides compared with dentate adults.[6,12] Nonstarch polysaccharide levels also have been shown to be lower in edentate adults than in dentate adults[9–14]; these same levels are reduced in patients who have difficulty chewing.[15] This is reflected in the Survey Europe on Nutrition in the Elderly: Concerted Action study, which investigated the dentition and dietary intake of the elderly in 12 European cities and the state of Connecticut in the United States. Edentulous patients were found to have more chewing difficulties; lower intakes of carbohydrates and vitamin B_6; and a trend toward reduced vitamins B_1 and C, fiber, calcium, and iron intake compared with dentate adults.[16]

Blood-derived values of key nutrients also appear to be influenced by oral health status. Data from the National Diet and Nutrition Survey (NDNS) conducted in elderly men and women from Great Britain showed that, even after controlling for confounding variables, plasma ascorbate and retinol were significantly associated with dental status. Furthermore, the relationship between ascorbate and tooth number was statistically significant. There also was a trend toward higher levels of most nutrients in dentate individuals. These findings are consistent with the results of the dietary intake of these populations.[13]

The effect of these findings perhaps is more clearly seen in the frail elderly. In a study reviewing the relationship between the oral and systemic health of institutionalized subjects, those with compromised oral function had both a significantly lower body mass index

Table 2-1 Change in food selection in patients treated with fixed or removable implant-supported prostheses

Food type	Preoperative*	Postoperative*	*P* value
Bread	20 (70)	18 (72)	.500
Cheese	10 (38)	20 (80)	.002
Carrots	2 (8)	13 (52)	.003
Apples	7 (30)	15 (60)	.035
Nuts	2 (8)	12 (48)	.006
Bacon	11 (42)	19 (76)	.021
Lettuce	22 (85)	22 (88)	.725

After Allen and McMillan.[22]

*The number and percentage (%) of subjects in each group who indicate they eat various foods.

(BMI) and low serum albumin concentration.[17] The presence of less than six occluding pairs of teeth was a strong predictor of malnutrition as determined by these parameters. A 6-year longitudinal study of the institutionalized elderly showed a greater decline in physical ability and higher mortality rates in edentulous subjects without dentures compared to patients with 20 or more teeth.[18]

Partially dentate patients with less than 10 occluding pairs of teeth have been shown to have undesirable nutrient intake both before and after rehabilitation. Patients with either a fixed or removable mandibular prosthesis who followed a diet low in nonstarch polysaccharides at baseline showed no significant improvement.[15] Other studies also have failed to show an increase in the intake of nonstarch polysaccharides following prosthetic rehabilitation.[19] It is, however, unlikely that, without restoring some function, patients would eat more challenging foods, and it therefore follows that high-quality restorations would help solve the problem of adequate nutritional intake for the edentulous elderly.

Implant-Supported Prostheses Versus Conventional Dentures

In a within-subject cross-over clinical trial, patients reported significantly less chewing difficulty with both fixed and removable implant-supported prostheses compared to their original dentures.[20] When examining mastication time and amplitude of masticatory strokes, the overdenture appeared to be no less efficient than the fixed prosthesis.[21]

A group of edentulous patients fitted with fixed or removable implant-supported prostheses reported an improvement in ability to chew hard and soft foods. At the conclusion of the study, there was a significant increase in the number of implant-restored patients who were able to eat a range of foods such as cheese, carrots, apples, nuts, and bacon; however, these improvements were not seen in the conventional denture groups[22] (Table 2-1).

In a randomized clinical trial comparing conventional dentures to implant-supported overdentures, implant treatment was significantly associated with lower posttreatment

Oral Health Impact Profile (OHIP) scores, which indicates a better quality of life.[23] In a second randomized clinical trial with patients aged 65 to 75 years, the implant-supported overdentures group reported a greater ability to chew tough meat and raw fruits and vegetables than the conventional denture group; results similar to the former study were found for quality of life (unpublished data).

Nutritional Status and Implant Prostheses

Although there is some evidence that patients can chew foods more easily and that there can be a change in eating patterns following provision of implant-supported prostheses, to date there has been no information suggesting that these improvements manifest themselves in changes to the patients' nutritional state. This hypothesis recently has been tested in a pilot study with patients provided with mandibular overdentures supported by two implants or conventional dentures at 6 months posttreatment.

Sixty independent male and female adults, aged 65 to 75 years, who responded to a newspaper advertisement were enrolled in the study. All subjects were required to have been edentulous for at least 5 years. Subjects were randomized and received either mandibular overdentures (n = 30) retained by ball attachments on two transmucosal implants (ITI 048.242/243, Straumann, Waldenburg, Switzerland) or conventional complete dentures (n = 30), both opposed by new conventional maxillary dentures. In addition to other data collected, assessments of nutritional states using 3-day food records, blood parameters, and anthropometric measurements were gathered at baseline, then at 6 and 12 months after delivery of the prostheses. Data were gathered by a research dietician and a

trained nurse who were blind to treatment assignment.

Height and weight were measured to calculate BMI. Skinfold thickness (SFT) was measured on the dominant side of the body in the biceps, triceps, and subscapular and suprailiac areas and the waist-to-hip ratio was determined. Other parameters measured included estimated percentage body fat and lean body mass by SFT, bioelectrical impedance analysis, and handgrip strength. Complete blood cell count, nutritional parameters, and nutrients, including albumin, pre-albumin, carotene, plasma cobalamin (vitamin B_{12}), serum and erythrocyte folate, and serum iron were determined from 40-mL blood samples. Data from the food diaries were analyzed using a proprietary software package. A history of gastrointestinal symptoms and self-reported measures of dietary habits also were recorded. Results at 6 months after delivery of the prosthesis are summarized below.

Dietary intake and habits

As in previous studies, no difference between groups was shown for nutrient intake using food diaries. By contrast, there was a significant improvement after treatment in the response of the conventional denture group for four questions regarding chewing difficulty. The implant group noted an improvement for 13 items also regarding chewing difficulty. The implant group was less limited in their choice of food and perceived less need to drink in order to swallow compared to their pretreatment abilities. They also reported significantly less difficulty chewing pieces of meat and whole, hard fruits and vegetables compared to their pretreatment ability to chew. A group of edentulous patients provided with fixed and removable implant-supported prostheses was reported to be able to eat a wider range of foods posttreatment[22]; this finding is echoed in this study in patients treated with removable mandibular overdentures supported by two implants. The foods enjoyed by patients post-treatment typically are major sources of vitamins, minerals, proteins, and fiber. In interviews and focus groups, the patients who were provided with implant-supported prostheses expressed a range of positive comments about their increased ability to eat, from being able to bite, chew, and talk without losing the dentures to savoring long-avoided foods such as steak and apples.

Anthropometric data

There was a significant improvement in the implant group at 6 months for a range of body composition and anthropometric measures, namely increased percentage body fat; increased SFT at the biceps, subscapular area, and abdomen; and significant decreases in waist circumference and the waist-to-hip ratio. In the conventional denture group, significant increases were found only for the biceps SFT. These results indicate a healthier distribution of adipose tissue in the implant patients since the increased percentage of fat was made of fat deposits outside of the abdominal region.

Blood nutrient data

The altered eating habits are reflected in the comparisons of blood parameters. A significant increase was seen for the concentration of serum albumin, hemoglobin, and vitamin B_{12}, with a trend toward increased carotene in the implant group. No significant changes were seen in the conventional denture group. In the implant group, serum albumin concentration increased significantly by 1.4 g/L, a similar difference to that found in elderly adults who regularly take dietary supplements.[24] Serum albumin is recognized as an indicator of general good health and nutritional status. Lower serum albumin levels are associated with a higher prevalence of cancer, cardiovascular disease, and mortality.[25]

Vitamin B_{12} deficiency is associated with both hematological (eg, megaloblastic anemia and bone marrow suppression) and neurological diseases (eg, peripheral neuropathy). It also is associated with increased plasma levels of homocysteine, a known risk factor for cardiovascular disease.[11] The significant increase in serum B_{12} concentration in the implant overdenture group, in combination with the increases in albumin and hemoglobin (iron), may be linked to the increased ability to chew meat. There were no significant changes in the blood parameters of the conventional denture group.

The dietary changes were not reflected in the nutritional intake calculated from the food diaries. Contrary to the blood nutrient data, nutritional intake assessment requires large numbers of patients to find differences due to the great interindividual variability in the reported intakes.

Summary

There is strong evidence to suggest that people with a reduction in tooth number are more likely to practice forms of food avoidance, especially when there are less than 10 occluding pairs of teeth. This food avoidance may lead patients to a dietary intake that falls short of the recommended amount of a wide range of nutrients.

Edentulous patients with fixed or removable implant prostheses have reported an improvement in their ability to chew foods. This also has been reflected in the number patients treated with implant-supported prostheses who report eating a wider range of foods. Preliminary results suggest that providing edentulous patients with one of the least complicated forms of implant prosthesis, the mandibular overdenture supported by two implants, improves their nutritional state at 6 months posttreatment. In addition to reporting a higher capacity to chew and bite hard foods, patients reported that they were less limited in food choice. Compared to the conventional denture group, the implant-supported overdenture group showed improvements in several blood parameters and anthropometric measures. These initial findings must be confirmed in a larger randomized clinical trial, but already may point to previously unknown advantages of implant-supported treatment.

Acknowledgments

This study was funded by University Industry grant No. UCT36052 from the Canadian Institutes of Health Research and Straumann Canada Limited. Dr Thomason is supported by grants from the PPP Foundation, United Kingdom, and the Ethicon Foundation Fund.

References

1. Bates JF, Stafford GD, Harrison A. Masticatory function—A review of the literature. III. Masticatory performance and efficiency. J Oral Rehabil 1976;3: 57–67.

2. Kayser AF. Shortened dental arches and oral function. J Oral Rehabil 1981;8:457–462.

3. Allen PF, Witter DF, Wilson NH, Kayser AF. Shortened dental arch therapy: Views of consultants in restorative dentistry in the United Kingdom. J Oral Rehabil 1996;23:481–485.

4. Steele JG, Ayatollahi SM, Walls AW, Murray JJ. Clinical factors related to reported satisfaction with oral function amongst dentate older adults in England. Community Dent Oral Epidemiol 1997;25:143–149.

5. Farrel J. The effect of mastication on the digestion of food. Br Dent J 1956;100:149–155.

6. Osterberg T, Steen B. Relationship between dental state and dietary intake in 70-year-old males and females in Goteborg, Sweden: A population study. J Oral Rehabil 1982;9:509–521.

7. Geissler CA, Bates JF. The nutritional effects of tooth loss. Am J Clin Nutr 1984;39:478–489.

8. Sheiham A, Steele JG, Marcenes W, Finch S, Walls AW. The impact of oral health on stated ability to eat certain foods; findings from the national diet and nutrition survey of older people in Great Britain. Gerodontology 1999;16:11–20.

9. Joshipura KJ, Willett WC, Douglass CW. The impact of edentulousness on food and nutrient intake. J Am Dent Assoc 1996;127:459–467.

10. Joshipura KJ, Hu FB, Manson JE, et al. The effect of fruit and vegetable intake on risk for coronary heart disease. Ann Intern Med 2001;134:1106–1114.

11. Boushey CJ, Beresford SA, Omenn GS, Motulsky AG. A quantitative assessment of plasma homocysteine as a risk factor for vascular disease. Probable benefits of increasing folic acid intakes. JAMA 1995; 274:1049–1057.

12. Hinds K, Gregory JR. National diet and nutrition survey: People aged 65 years or over. Vol 2: Report of the oral health survey. London: Stationary Office, 1998.

13. Sheiham A, Steele JG, Marcenes W, et al. The relationship among dental status, nutrient intake, and nutritional status in older people. J Dent Res 2001; 80:408–413.

14. Moynihan PJ, Snow S, Jepson NJ, Butler TJ. Intake of non-starch polysaccharide (dietary fibre) in edentulous and dentate persons: An observational study. Br Dent J 1994;177:243–247.

15. Moynihan PJ, Butler TJ, Thomason JM, Jepson NJ. Nutrient intake in partially dentate patients: The effect of prosthetic rehabilitation. J Dent 2000;28: 557–563.

16. Fontijn-Tekamp FA, van't Hof MA, Slagter AP, van Waas MA. The state of dentition in relation to nutrition in elderly Europeans in the SENECA study of 1993. Eur J Clin Nutr 1996;50:S117–S122.

17. Mojon P, Budtz-Jorgensen E, Rapin CH. Relationship between oral health and nutrition in very old people. Age Ageing 1999;28:463–468.

18. Shimazaki Y, Soh I, Saito T, et al. Influence of dentition status on physical disability, mental impairment, and mortality in institutionalized elderly people. J Dent Res 2001;80:340–345.

19. Sebring NG, Guckes AD, Li SH, McCarthy GR. Nutritional adequacy of reported intake of edentulous subjects treated with new conventional or implant-supported mandibular dentures. J Prosthet Dent 1995;74:358–363.

20. de Grandmont P, Feine JS, Tache R, et al. Within-subject comparisons of implant-supported mandibular prostheses: Psychometric evaluation. J Dent Res 1994;73:1096–1104.

21. Feine JS, Maskawi K, de Grandmont P, Donohue WB, Tanguay R, Lund JP. Within-subject comparisons of implant-supported mandibular prostheses: Evaluation of masticatory function. J Dent Res 1994;73: 1646–1656.

22. Allen PF, McMillan AS. Food selection and perceptions of chewing ability following provision of implant and conventional prostheses in complete denture wearers. Clin Oral Implants Res 2002;13: 320–326.

23. Awad MA, Locker D, Korner-Bitensky N, Feine JS. Measuring the effect of intra-oral implant rehabilitation on health-related quality of life in a randomized controlled clinical trial. J Dent Res 2000;79: 1659–1663.

24. de Jong N, Paw MJ, de Groot LC, de Graaf C, Kok FJ, van Staveren WA. Functional biochemical and nutrient indices in frail elderly people are partly affected by dietary supplements but not by exercise. J Nutr 1999;129:2028–2036.

25. Phillips A, Shaper AG, Whincup PH. Association between serum albumin and mortality from cardiovascular disease, cancer, and other causes. Lancet 1989;2:1434–1436.

CHAPTER 3

The Impact of Edentulism on Function and Quality of Life

Michael I. MacEntee

A recent analysis of information collected by the author and his colleagues in Vancouver, British Columbia, revealed that older adults who believe that dentistry is usually painful, or who expect to lose all of their natural teeth, are about three times more likely to report 5 years later that they are dissatisfied with life. Although this does not prove a cause-effect relationship between poor dental beliefs or expectations and poor quality of life (QOL), it does suggest an association. Chapter 1 noted that the prevalence of edentulism dropped by approximately 10% for each decade of the past 30 years in the United States, yet, because of population growth, especially in older age groups, there will be an increase in the number edentulous patients who have no natural teeth in one or both arches. Hence, the need for dentures will not diminish over the next quarter century and those in most need of dentures are most likely to be among society's poorest and least advantaged.

Chronic disability now is the major health care challenge of Western society. Consequently, with society's prolonged life expectancy, there is growing interest in QOL and sensitivity to the "lived experiences" of chronic illness.[1] The World Health Organization (WHO) expressed the importance of this sensitivity in 1948 by recognizing health as more than simply the absence of disease and noting that healthy societies have a complicated mixture of social, economic, and cultural characteristics. Edentulism is a prevalent disability with all the characteristics of a chronic illness. It is incurable and functionally and psychologically disruptive. It carries with it a social stigma, and it requires specific management strategies to overcome or limit its disruptive effects.[2]

Impact of Edentulism on Function

Mandibular Function

It is widely agreed in clinical discourse that the dentition or, more particularly, the occlusal arrangement of teeth has no direct relationship to the functional health of the temporomandibular joint, other than in extremely unusual situations. The possibility of a dysfunctional relationship has been the source of a long and agonizing debate with serious treatment implications. Studies on the distribution and management of mandibular dysfunction have been hampered generally by disagreements over the validity and reliability of diagnostic criteria or clinical assessments.[3] There are reports of chronically abnormal jaw movements attributed to tooth loss and denture use, but the evidence rests heavily on the identification and interpretation of dysfunction.[4] For example, researchers typically identify jaw dysfunction if the maximum separation of a patient's maxillary and mandibular incisor teeth is less than 40 mm, yet there is no empirical evidence that patients are impaired or even inconvenienced by this limited jaw movement.[3] Indeed, many complete denture wearers probably limit tooth separation and jaw movements consciously or subconsciously to stabilize and control their dentures. Certainly, stress-induced clenching can damage the denture-supporting mucosa; however, the jaw and temporomandibular joint of most edentulous denture wearers seem to move without restriction or discomfort.

Denture-Induced Mucosal Disorders

Most denture wearers, especially men, have some clinical evidence of denture-induced stomatitis, denture-related hyperplasia, angular cheilitis, or inflammation of the denture-supporting mucosa. Surprisingly, evidence shows that denture quality does not seem to have much influence on the prevalence of these disorders.[5] There also is evidence that the risk of oral cancer is elevated synergistically in denture wearers who drink alcohol excessively and who smoke tobacco. Nonetheless, the incidence of oral cancer for edentulous patients is very small, and most of the denture-related pathoses are relatively innocuous inflammatory responses in the mucosa.

Denture-Induced Residual Ridge Resorption

The residual ridge supporting a complete denture is inherently unstable due to unpredictable resorption and remodeling of the alveolar bone when natural teeth are removed.[6] Consequently, resorption of the residual ridge disturbs the comfort and retention of a denture, which, in turn, can irritate the peripheral mucosa to produce an epulis fissuratum.[7] The influence of dentures on the supporting jawbone is unclear. Denture base pressure, especially if it is unevenly distributed on the residual ridge, infected, or structurally defective, can precipitate a low-grade inflammation of the supporting mucosa and the underlying bone,[8] but usually the damage is reversible.[9] Clinical experience reveals that the discomfort of an ill-fitting complete denture, especially in the mandible, can be very difficult for the denture wearer to manage. A mandibular residual ridge provides a complete denture with less than one quarter of the support offered by the periodontium to natural teeth, yet some patients expect the prosthesis to replace natural teeth in every respect. Obviously, this expectation is unrealistic and many denture wearers cannot cope with their dentures, no matter how well they have been made.[10]

Use of Dental Services

The absence of teeth is a principal reason given by the edentate for not visiting a dentist regularly, and patterns of attendance for preventive health care established during youth seem to continue into old age.[11–13] In general, people seek medical attention because they perceive that something is wrong, rather than because they detect an objective clinical sign or symptom, and "wrongness" is relative to other people in similar circumstances. Elderly denture wearers, for example, make little effort to seek dental care probably because they are surrounded by peers who accept tooth loss and discomfort from dentures with resignation.

Food Selection, Mastication, and Diet

Numerous studies have been conducted on food choices of people with or without natural teeth (see chapter 2), but little attention has been paid to the relationship between the adaptive and coping skills of edentulous individuals and the food they eat. For example, a recent study in the United Kingdom revealed that edentulous older adults with uncomfortable and well-worn complete dentures noted difficulty eating some foods, although most of the group ate nearly all of the food available to them despite difficulties chewing.[14] Two thirds of the participants expressed no regrets about this difficulty or impairment, possibly because they managed to adapt and cope successfully with their impairment without undue distress. So, even in this select group of older adults, there was little demand for other prostheses to enhance food selection and mastication. A much larger population-based investigation in the United Kingdom found that edentulous older adults avoided some foods, notably fruit, vegetables, and other dietary fibers.[15] One tenth of the edentulous participants interviewed said that 10 of the 16 food types assessed were difficult to eat, and blood tests revealed that they had significantly lower levels of plasma ascorbate and plasma retinol compared to dentulous participants. Therefore, edentulism appears to increase the risk of dermatological and visual problems in aging adults.

There is evidence elsewhere[16] that poor chewing ability is one of several predictors of involuntary weight loss in old age. Food processing and preparation offers the possibility of a varied and nutritious diet, even in the absence of teeth, although a distasteful, unattractive, or bland diet predisposes edentulous adults to avoidance and malnutrition, and almost certainly disturbs quality of life. Eating is one of the more enduring and attainable pleasures in life, even when patients face declining health and disability, and people with poor teeth or ill-fitting dentures are at particular risk of undernourishment if they dislike eating mashed foods.[17] Overall, it is clear that edentulous people without dentures or those with dentures that are loose, unstable, or painful restrict their selection of nutritious foods.

Social Interactions

An edentulous person carries the label "toothless" or "denture wearer" along with the associated stigma of social embarrassment, which can potentially lead to social avoidance and isolation that are characteristic of chronic illness.[18,19] Social embarrassment from denture use is more likely among younger adults for whom complete edentulism is the exception, but it can embarrass older adults also, especially in Western cultures where a perfect smile and the appearance of youth are almost prerequisites for social and commercial success. Complete dentures today, in contrast to half a century ago, are almost synonymous with poverty and personal neglect.

Tooth loss can cause profound and lasting psychologic disturbances. Fiske et al[20] used a narrative analysis of transcripts from open-ended interviews to provide one of the few systematically obtained insights into the range of feelings about edentulism among complete denture patients attending a dental school clinic. They discovered that tooth loss, like the loss of other important parts of the body or the death of a friend, precipitated bereavement, reduction of self-confidence, disturbance of self-image, shame, and secrecy. As with other events, bereavement for lost teeth proceeds through the predictable stages of denial, anger, depression, adaptation, and acceptance. Some denture wearers never get over the anger and depression associated with the indignity of tooth loss, and they become very disturbed by chronic self-conscious feelings of being "a lesser person" with a disfigured and unattractive appearance. In a different qualitative investigation of the significance of the mouth to older adults, a woman explained that "You want to have nice teeth, [because] that's the basis of your good looks" and "I never go anywhere without my teeth, I just feel terrible without teeth."[21] These statements clearly indicate that teeth are a major medium of emotional expression and a focus of self. Moreover, an enormous psychologic burden is placed on complete denture wearers in contemporary culture, with its emphasis on personal grooming, fitness, and youth.

Impact of Edentulism on Quality of Life

Defining Oral Health–Related Quality of Life

Teeth influence function, and missing teeth can be disabling within the functional context of personal appearance, appetite, breath odor, eating, general health, mood, recreation, sexual activity, weight, and work.[20–23] However, theories supporting relationships between functional disability, health perceptions, and QOL are vague,[24] in part because the point of personal reference for QOL changes constantly.[25] There are several questionnaires available for collecting information on the functional and psychologic effects of tooth loss and dental

disorder,[26] although the validity of the connection between measures of functional impairment and QOL is doubtful.[1,24,25,27] There is a growing sense that health-related QOL and disability are better interpreted than measured.[1,21,24] In any event, for most adults, QOL is good when biological and social needs are satisfied. Typically, adults are motivated to identify these needs in the context of safety and belonging, in addition to love, self-esteem, and self-actualization.[28] In dental terms, perhaps this means that adults are motivated to enhance QOL by replacing missing teeth when physical pressures (eg, tough foods) threaten the physiological drive to eat, or when social (eg, cosmetic) pressures disturb either self-esteem or the ability to succeed in life. The attributes of QOL are evolving constantly; however, they affect adults in at least four prominent dimensions: (1) psychologic health and function; (2) socioeconomic status; (3) life satisfaction; and (4) self-esteem.[27]

Psychologic Health and Function

Disability results as much from social and environmental pressures as it does from physical impairment. Intolerance to dentures, for example, is influenced more by stigma than by the severity of residual ridge resorption. Similarly, the depression and social isolation induced by chronic orofacial pain or by dental disfigurement are much more disabling than the painful stimuli or the dysfunctional arrangement of the teeth. On the other hand, people who have a strong sense of coherence choose to adapt and cope with unstable, unsightly, and painful dentures by using psychosocial buffers that help them to accept their impairments.[29] Nonetheless, some complete denture wearers are tormented by fears of embarrassment and rejection and see dentures as a reflection of personal decline.

Socioeconomic Status

Edentulism is becoming a disorder of the poor, who are the least adept at coping with health problems, whereas more educated and financially secure adults are informed of health care options and can afford the necessary professional care.[13] In 1995, 36% of single persons and 14% of families—17% of the total Canadian population—had income levels below the poverty line. One perspective defines poverty as a lack of resources "for achieving self-respect, taking part in the life of the community, (and) appearing in public without shame."[30] The consequences, of course, are that patients with little money cannot afford preventive dental treatment; they are ill-informed to prevent tooth loss and therefore end up feeling ashamed about their complete dentures.

Life Satisfaction and Self-esteem

Self-assessments of health and life satisfaction, especially by older adults, typically are much more positive than the ratings made by the clinicians.[13] In contrast, functional disorders of any kind, including uncomfortable or unstable dentures, are associated with poor life satisfaction, which perhaps discourages some denture wearers from seeking treatment altogether.[12] *Self-esteem* is a descriptive term by which we identify ourselves in contrast to our aspirations, or judge ourselves in response to social interactions. It is a dominant theme for many denture wearers who struggle with concerns of attractiveness and normality related to the appearance and stability of their dentures. There is little or no empirical evidence that self-esteem or the lack of it is an enduring trait. Even so, it is possible for a patient with a well-established low self-esteem about his or her dental appearance to remain resistant to treatment, no matter how heroic or technically sound it may be. Clearly, this possibility has important implications for denture and oral implant–related treatments. In any case, it is reasonable to assume that denture wearers who are very concerned about their dentures, in contrast to those who are less concerned, are more likely to experience a relatively poor QOL. In fact, patients usually are motivated to obtain oral implants due to the discomfort, insecurity, and overall dissatisfaction with conventional dentures. There is ample clinical and behavioral evidence that implant-supported dentures are much more satisfying to patients than conventional dentures, perhaps because the implant denture feels more like an integral part of the body.[31]

Summary

With prolonged life expectancy, chronic illness is the major health care problem in Western society. Consequently, management rather than cure of chronic disorders is a primary challenge facing all health care professions. Social labels and stigmas influence tooth loss like other chronic disabilities that disturb physiologic and psychosocial function substantially. Fortunately, most complete denture wearers are able to adapt and cope with their disability effectively without much disturbance to their quality of life. Nonetheless, other denture wearers suffer substantially from chronic dysfunction, pain, low self-esteem, and reduced quality of life. For these patients, dentures supported by implants, especially in the mandible, would offer relief, comfort, and optimism.

References

1. Bury M. Illness narratives: Fact or fiction? Sociol Health Illn 2001;25:263–285.
2. Locker D. Disability and Disadvantage: The Consequences of Chronic Illness. London: Tavistock Publications, 1983.
3. MacEntee MI, Weiss R, Waxler-Morrison NE, Morrison BJ. Mandibular dysfunction in an institutionalized and predominantly elderly population. J Oral Rehabil 1987;14:523–529.
4. Dworkin SF, LeResche L. Research diagnostic criteria for temporomandibular disorders: Review, criteria, examinations and specifications, critique. J Craniomandib Disord 1992;6:301–355.
5. MacEntee MI, Glick N, Stolar E. Age, gender, dentures and oral mucosal disorders. Oral Diseases 1998;4:32–36.
6. Tallgren A. The continuing reduction of the residual alveolar ridges in complete denture wearers: A mixed longitudinal study covering 25 years. J Prosthet Dent 1972;27:120–132.
7. MacEntee MI. The prevalence of edentulism and diseases related to dentures. A literature review. J Oral Rehabil 1985;12:195–207.
8. Lytle RB. Complete denture construction based on a study of the deformation of the underlying soft tissues. J Prosthet Dent 1959;9:539–551.
9. Sharry JJ. Complete Denture Prosthodontics, ed 3. New York: McGraw-Hill, 1974.
10. Zarb GA, Bolender CL, Carlsson GE (eds). Prosthodontic Treatment for Edentulous Patients. St. Louis: Mosby, 1997:3-7.
11. Slade GD, Locker D, Leake JL, Wu ASM, Dunkley G. The oral health, status and treatment needs of adults aged 65+ living independently in Ottawa-Carleton. Can J Public Health 1990;81:114–119.
12. MacEntee MI, Hill PM, Wong G, Mojon P, Berkowitz J, Glick N. Predicting concerns for oral health among institutionalized elders. J Public Health Dent 1991;51:82–91.
13. MacEntee MI, Stolar E, Glick N. The influence of age and gender on oral health and related behaviour in an independent elderly population. Community Dent Oral Epidemiol 1993;21:234–239.
14. Millwood J, Heath MR. Food choice by older people: The use of semi-structured interviews with open and closed questions. Gerodontology 2000;17:25–32.
15. Sheiham A, Steele J. Does the condition of the mouth and teeth affect the ability to eat certain foods, nutrient and dietary intake and nutritional status amongst older people? Public Health Nutr 2001; 4:797–803.
16. Sullivan D, Walls R, Lipschitz D. Protein-energy undernutrition and the risk of mortality within 1 year of hospital discharge in a select population of geriatric rehabilitation patients. Am J Clin Nutr 1991; 43:559–605.
17. Lamy M, Mojon P, Kalykakis G, Legrand R, Budtz-Jorgensen E. Oral status and nutrition in the institutionalized elderly. J Dent 1999;27:443–448.
18. Scheff TJ. The labeling of mental illness. Am Soc Rev 1974;39:444–452.
19. Goffma E. Stigma: Notes on the Management of Spoiled Identity. Englewood Cliffs, NJ: Prentice Hall, 1963.
20. Fiske J, Davis DM, Frances C, Gelbier S. The emotional effects of tooth loss in edentulous people. Br Dent J 1998;184:90–93.
21. MacEntee MI, Hole R, Stolar E. The significance of the mouth in old age. Soc Sci Med 1997;45:1449–1458.
22. Strauss RP, Hunt RJ. Understanding the value of teeth to older adults: Influences on quality of life. J Am Dent Assoc 1993;124:105–110.
23. Anttila SS, Knuuttilka MLE, Sakki TK. Relationship of depressive symptoms to edentulousness, dental health, and dental health behavior. Acta Odontol Scand 2001;59:406–412.
24. Hunt SM. The problem of quality of life. Quality Life Res 1997;6:205–212.
25. Allison PJ, Locker D, Feine JS. Quality of life: A dynamic construct. Soc Sci Med 1997;45:221–230.
26. Slade G (ed). Measuring Oral Health and Quality of Life. Chapel Hill, NC: University of North Carolina Press, 1997.
27. George LK, Bearon LB. Quality of Life in Older Persons: Meaning and Measurement. New York: Human Science Press, 1980.
28. Maslow AH. Motivation and Personality, ed 2. New York: Harper & Row, 1970:35–47.
29. Stolar GE, MacEntee MI, Hill P. Seniors' assessment of their own health: The case for contextual evaluation. Int J Aging Hum Dev 1992;35:305–317.
30. Sen Amartya . Developments as Freedom. Oxford: Oxford University Press, 1999:73–75.
31. MacEntee MI, Walton JN. The economics of complete dentures and implant-related services: A framework for analysis and preliminary outcomes. J Prosthet Dent 1998;79:24–30.

CHAPTER 4

Patient Preferences and Expectations

Manal A. Awad

For treatment evaluation, patient self-perceived health and treatment satisfaction are used to measure outcome effectiveness. These values are usually referred to as *patient-based measures* because they are based on patients' treatment perceptions.[1–3] In the last decade, more studies have measured patients' perceptions of oral prostheses, including implant-supported overdentures, rather than solely considering clinical outcomes such as survival rates of implants and anatomical changes. While satisfactory clinical outcomes are important factors in the evaluation of the effectiveness of implant overdentures, these outcomes involve only the technical aspect of the prostheses. Consequently, they do not reflect the patient's opinion and degree of satisfaction with the treatment. This is an important aspect to consider, as edentulism is a chronic condition and therapy is palliative, aimed at improving function and quality of life.[1]

The patient's point of view is important in light of reported results that show a poor association between patients' satisfaction with their prosthesis and the clinical qualities of the prosthesis as assessed by the clinicians.[4–9] For

example, reports show that, although there is a weak association between patient satisfaction and clinical evaluation of the denture fit, there is a stronger association between patients' perceived masticatory ability and satisfaction with their prostheses.[9] Similar findings suggest that laboratory results of masticatory efficiency, rather than patient satisfaction ratings, should determine the presence of denture problems. Other findings have suggested that masticatory efficiency tests were poor predictors of patients' choice of prostheses; however, satisfaction ratings of different treatment aspects, such as comfort and stability, were associated with patient preferences. Furthermore, most studies that attempted to correlate patient satisfaction ratings of treatment and the clinician's opinion of the same treatment have found these correlations to be poor[8]; also, clinicians' ratings were not predictive of patient satisfaction. These discrepancies were attributed to the fact that clinicians usually apply predetermined criteria to their treatment evaluation that do not take into consideration the behavioral and psychosocial impact of therapy. For these reasons, there has been considerable interest in understanding and evaluating patients' preferences, expectations, and perceived ability to function with oral prostheses.

Patient Preferences

There is an increased appreciation among the medical community for the need to incorporate patient preferences into the medical decision-making process. This necessity came about as a result of the dramatic shift toward patient-centered care, in which health care is suited to patients' long-term needs.[10] Health care providers' interest has broadened beyond survival into the areas of psychosocial function and perceived health; in fact, it is believed that when patients participate in decisions regarding their health care, they tend to respond better to treatment.[11] Patient-based measures, such as quality of life, become an important outcome of treatment.[1]

Better understanding of patient preferences and the possible consequence of treatment satisfaction can be important in predicting patient behaviors, including demand for particular services.

Definition

It is possible for patients to prefer one form of therapy over another, not because they believe the outcome is more favorable, but instead because they find the process to be more acceptable. For example, patients may prefer to receive conventional dentures rather than implant-supported prostheses because of a fear of surgery; the decision is based on fear rather than a belief that conventional dentures provide the same stability as do implant-supported overdentures. Therefore, the term *preference* should be used with a clear understanding of what the prosthesis does and does not in-

clude.[12] Preference should be distinguished from what the patient desires or wants because of reasons not necessarily related to the treatment. In clinical practice, associated preferences should be based on estimated risks and benefits of proposed treatments with known efficacy. Patients do not make decisions based solely on choices that fulfill an immediate or temporary need. This can be remedied through proper patient-clinician communication, including informing patients of possible outcomes of all available therapies; ideally then patients use this information in the decision-making process.

Evaluation

Incorporation of patient preferences in decision making is not uncommon in medicine. Patient preferences have been evaluated in studies of cancer,[13] arthritis,[14] and diabetes.[15] Results indicate that, given sufficient information, patients were able to make a decision regarding their choice of treatment. It also has been reported that patients who chose their treatment reported less pain compared to other patients who were not given this option.[11]

In dentistry, however, the role of patient preferences is rarely evaluated. Nevertheless, it is an important issue, especially in cases of oral rehabilitation in which patients are expected to live with the treatment for long periods of time.[2] In addition, patients' perceptions may influence their level of satisfaction with the prostheses and consequently impact quality of life.

In a within-subject cross-over clinical trial[16] comparing fixed and removable implant-supported prostheses, 15 patients were randomly divided into two groups. One group received a fixed prosthesis while the other group received a removable prosthesis. After a 2-month period of adaptation, the patients rated their prostheses. The current prostheses were then replaced with one of the other type so that each patient could rate both types of prosthesis, and the procedure was repeated. At the end of the trial, patients were given the opportunity to choose their preferred prostheses. Eight patients preferred the fixed prostheses and the other seven preferred the removable prostheses. Those patients who chose the fixed prostheses indicated that the most important factor governing their choice was stability; those who preferred the removable prostheses indicated that ease of cleaning was the most important factor. Eighteen months later all patients reported to be very satisfied with their choice, and 69% of the subjects gave the same reasons that they had given earlier for their choice. These findings suggest that patients' preferences were not arbitrary, but instead reflected what they perceived to be important characteristics of the prostheses. Nevertheless, patients in this study tried both treatments and their choice was made based on their own experience. In clinical practice, patients usually do not have such an opportunity, and preference for one form of treatment is determined by their current oral status and possible deficiencies that may exist in their dentures.

The association between patient preferences and satisfaction with their current conventional dentures was evaluated in a randomized clinical trial[17] comparing mandibular implant overdentures and conventional dentures among 136 edentulous patients (aged 35 to 65 years) seeking replacement of their current prostheses. These patients responded to questionnaires regarding their satisfaction level with their current prostheses. In addition, patients were asked to indicate which treatment they preferred when given a choice. The results showed that 79% of patients expressed a treatment preference, of which 60% preferred

implant-supported prostheses and 19% preferred conventional dentures. When patients later were asked about the reasons for their preferences, those who preferred implant prostheses indicated that they wanted stable, comfortable prostheses and to have less bone loss. Patients who opted for conventional dentures explained that they were afraid of the surgery itself, possible complications, and the inconvenience associated with these factors. Among the patients who preferred implants, 71% were aged 50 years and older, as were 58% of those who preferred conventional dentures. Further analysis revealed that women showed a greater preference for conventional dentures compared to men ($P = .08$). As hypothesized, patients who were dissatisfied with their conventional dentures were significantly more likely to prefer implant treatment ($P < .05$). In fact, relatively higher satisfaction ratings were significantly associated with less preference for implants (Table 4-1). However, posttreatment satisfaction ratings for conventional dentures and implant-supported prostheses showed patients' treatment preferences were not significant predictors of posttreatment satisfaction ratings or quality-of-life ratings. These findings suggest that, irrespective of patients' treatment preferences, those who received the implant prostheses were significantly more satisfied with the function of their prostheses and that they also experienced significantly fewer oral health–related quality of life problems compared to those who received conventional dentures.

The fact that there was no strong evidence for the effects of initial preference on end satisfaction with oral prostheses in this clinical trial should not be interpreted to mean that such effects of preference do not exist. It is possible that for this study the number of subjects recruited was not large enough to measure this association. Also, pa-

Table 4-1 Patient characteristics associated with prosthesis preference

Variables	Conventional treatment			Implant treatment		
	OR*[†]	95% CI	P value	OR*[‡]	95% CI	P value
Gender						
Men[§]						
Women	2.86	0.89, 4.82	.08	1.86	0.69, 4.9	.23
Age						
< 50 years[§]						
≥ 50 years	1.43	0.44, 4.66	.54	2.33	0.88, 6.23	.09
Education level						
Low[§]						
High	0.18	0.04, 0.77	.02	0.20	0.05, 0.76	.02
Level of satisfaction[‖]						
Low (0–25 mm)[§]						
Medium (26–75 mm)	0.41	0.10, 1.67	.22	0.31	0.09, 0.96	.05
High (76–100 mm)	0.36	0.08, 1.54	.17	0.11	0.03, 0.41	.001

Data from Awad et al.[17]
*Multivariate odds ratios (OR) were estimated from polytomous logistic regression including all the above variables, using neutrality as reference outcome category.
[†]Estimated ORs for preference for conventional treatment.
[‡]Estimated ORs for preference for implant treatment.
[§]Reference category.
[‖]Satisfaction was rated on a 100-mm visual analog scale.

tient preferences could be a complex phenomena that may not be captured by one question; for even among those patients who prefer the same treatment, the strength of that preference may be different.[18] Consequently, the impact of patient preferences on satisfaction level and quality of life will not be the same. It would be helpful to both patients and clinicians to design questionnaires that ask patients about their preferences as well as measure the strength of those preferences. These instruments would enable clinicians to gain better understanding of the patient's point of view.

Clearly more research is needed to understand the reasons for patient preferences and the factors associated with those choices. For example, patients may prefer conventional dentures because of the inconveniences associated with implant insertion, such as pain, and they may even overestimate its duration. Research also shows, however, that patients who received implants experienced the most pain on the day of surgery, after which there was a

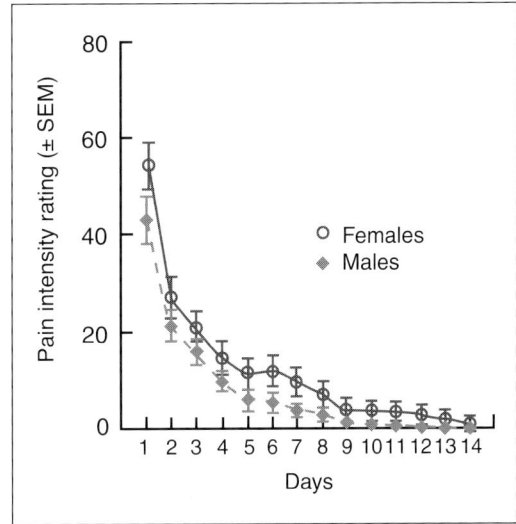

Fig 4-1 Pain intensity ratings according to gender. (Adapted with permission from Morin et al.[19])

continuous decline in reported pain (Fig 4-1). Clarification of such misconceptions would allow the distinction between those who believe in the efficacy of conventional dentures and others who want to avoid the possible side effects of implant overdentures.

Patient Expectations

Patient expectations of the outcome may play an important role in their preferences.[20] Unrealistic expectations may cause dramatic disappointment on the patient's behalf that may lead to negative consequences in making a treatment choice. Literature that examined the effect of expectations on treatment outcomes involved the study of placebo effect. Patients who experience the placebo effect may undergo symptomatic and physiologic changes when they believe they are receiving an effec-

tive treatment when, in fact, they are receiving an inert treatment. Studies measuring the clinical treatment outcome acknowledge that patient expectations play an important role on the outcome; however, the placebo effect is regarded as a factor that should be controlled rather than examined.

Some studies[21] attempt to explain the mechanism by which expectations can affect the outcome: (1) trigger of a physiologic response; (2) patient motivation to achieve better outcomes; (3) psychologic patient conditioning to observe certain symptoms and ignore others; and (4) changing of conceptions about the disease. It also has been suggested that patients who actively participate in their health care are better able to cope with their condition or treatment because they also try harder to experience successful outcomes and therefore achieve them. Others have suggested that patients with positive expectations tend to ig-

Table 4-2 Comparison of patients' expectation ratings on 100-mm visual analog scale for conventional dentures (CD) and implant overdentures (IO) according to preferences*

Preference	Expectations	Adults (35–65 y)			Seniors (65–75 y)		
		n	Mean	SD	n	Mean	SD
Conventional	CD	16	84.1	17	16	87.7	25.0
	IO	(16%)	83.8	18.5	(27%)	83.3	26.5
Implant	CD	62	79.8[†]	23.2	22	73.0[†]	30.0
	IO	(61%)	92.7	9.4	(45.0%)	94.8	6.8
Neutral	CD	24	87.8[†]	14.0	17	89.1	21.3
	IO	(23%)	92.4	12.1	(28.0%)	96.7	3.2

*Paired t test.
[†]Significant differences, P < .05.

nore adverse symptoms and concentrate on perceived improvements.[20] Moreover, expectations are related to the patient's level of knowledge and understanding of his or her condition which, in turn, affects his or her perceptions after receiving treatment. For example, it is unrealistic for edentulous patients to expect the performance of implant-supported prostheses to be identical to that of natural teeth. Such expectations may cause dramatic disappointment on the patient's behalf, which may lead to low treatment satisfaction. In addition, patients who experience a high level of anxiety toward the surgical procedure associated with the implants could be more sensitive to pain and focus on unfavorable symptoms. To the contrary, positive expectations may cause a reduction in anxiety and could lead to reports of more improvements and less adverse symptoms.

In two consecutive clinical trials with two groups of patients (adult group, aged 35 to 65 years, and senior group, aged 65 to 75 years), patient expectations for different oral pros-

theses (mandibular implant-supported overdentures and conventional dentures) were evaluated.[22] The results of both trials showed patients who preferred implant treatment had significantly higher expectations for this treatment than for the conventional treatment.[22] Those patients who preferred conventional dentures, however, did not rate their expectations for this treatment significantly higher than for implant overdentures (Table 4-2). The evaluation of the relationship between pretreatment expectations and posttreatment ratings of implant overdentures suggests that patients in the senior group found the treatment less satisfactory than they expected, although the finding is not significant, and patients in the adult group found the treatment exceeded their expectations (Table 4-3). Conventional dentures did not meet patients' expectations, even among those who preferred this treatment modality.

These findings indicate that, although some patients believe implant-supported prostheses could provide them with much more stability

Table 4-3 Comparison of patients' posttreatment expectations and satisfaction on 100-mm visual analog scale according to treatment received*

Treatment	Patient perception	Adults (35–65 y)			Seniors (65–75 y)		
		n	Mean	SD	n	Mean	SD
Conventional dentures	Expectation	47	85.8[†]	15.4	29	78.7[†]	29.8
	Satisfaction		64.5	34.7		60.8	31.8
Implant overdentures	Expectation	51	89.7	14.9	30	92.3	15.0
	Satisfaction		92.7	13.0		82.1	21.8

*Paired t test.
[†]Significant differences, P < .05.

and comfort, as well as an improved ability to chew, patients may still choose conventional treatment, most likely due to other factors that are important to them. This confirms earlier suggestions that patient preferences can be guided by factors other than the efficacy of the treatment, such as avoidance of surgery and surgical complications. Another possible explanation is that some patients who have worn conventional dentures for a long period of time may be skeptical about change and prefer to continue using the familiar treatment.[22]

The manner in which information is provided to patients regarding treatment options is important because it can heighten expectations, especially with respect to a new treatment such as implant overdentures. One possible solution is to introduce patients who seek this treatment modality to others who have experienced the intended prosthesis for a period of time; in this manner, expectations could be moderated.[22]

Summary

Patients should be informed that, to date, there is no evidence that implant-supported prostheses can restore oral function to the extent of the patient's own natural teeth. However, with proper communication, clinicians can discuss with patients their individual needs, and patients can reach a decision about the most appropriate and suitable treatment modality—from both a clinical and personal perspective. Some patients' main interest is a more stable prosthesis; these patients would be satisfied with a hybrid overdenture. On the other hand, a fixed prosthesis could be recommended to those who are seeking a denture that feels like a more natural part of their body.[22] Development of screening tools that identify those patients who have been significantly affected by tooth loss could be helpful, and if necessary, counseling could be provided. This may reduce unrealistic expectations that cannot be met.

References

1. Locker D. Patient-based assessments of the outcomes of implant therapy: A review of the literature. Int J Prosthodont 1998;11:453–461.

2. Awad MA, Feine JS. Measuring patient satisfaction with mandibular prostheses. Community Dent Oral Epidemiol 1998;26:400–405.

3. Weaver M, Patrik DL, Markson LE, et al. Patient satisfaction. Am J Manag Care 1997;3:579–594.

4. Smith M. Measurement of personality traits and their relationship to patient satisfaction with complete dentures. J Prosthet Dent 1976;35:492–503.

5. Berg E. The influence of some anamnestic, demographic and clinical variables on patient acceptance of new complete dentures. Acta Odontol Scand 1984;42:119–127.

6. Magnusson T. Clinical judgment and patients' evaluation of complete dentures five years after treatment. A follow-up study. Swed Dent J 1985;10:29–35.

7. Heyink JW, Heezen JH, Schaub RMH. Dentists' and patients' appraisal of complete dentures in a Dutch elderly population. Community Dent Oral Epidemiol 1986;14:323–326.

8. van Waas MAJ. The influence of clinical variables on patients' satisfaction with complete dentures. J Prosthet Dent 1990;63:307–310.

9. Langer A, Michman J, Seifert I. Factors influencing satisfaction with complete dentures in geriatric patients. J Prosthet Dent 1961;11:1019–1031.

10. Feine JS, Awad MA, Lund JP. The impact of patient preference on the design and interpretation of clinical trials. Community Dent Oral Epidemiol 1998;26:70–74.

11. Henshaw RC, Naji SA, Russel T, Tempeton AA. Comparison of medical abortion with surgical vacuum aspiration: Women's preferences and acceptability of treatment. Br Med J;307:714–717.

12. Till JE, Sutherland HJ, Meslin EM. Is there a role for preference assessments in research on quality of life oncology? Quality Life Research 1992;1:31–40.

13. Hack TF, Degner LF, Dyck DG. Relationship between preferences for decisional control and illness information among women with breast cancer: A quantitative analysis. Soc Sci Med 1994;39:279–289.

14. Kassirer J. Incorporation of patients' preferences into medical decisions. N Engl J Med 1994;330:1895–1896.

15. Bradley C. Designing medical and educational intervention studies. Diabetes Care 1993;16:509–518.

16. Feine JS, de Grandomont de P, Boudrias P, la Marche C, Tache R, Lund JP. Within-subject comparisons of implant-supported mandibular prostheses: Choice of prostheses. J Dent Res 1994;73:1105–1111.

17. Awad MA, Shapiro SH, Lund JP, Feine JS. Determinants of patients' treatment preferences in a clinical trial. Community Dent Oral Epidemiol 2000;28:119–125.

18. Desbiens NA, Muller-Rizner N, Hamel MB, Connors AF. Preferences for comfort care does not affect the pain experience of seriously ill patients. J Pain Symptom Manage 1998;16:281–289.

19. Morin C, Lund JP, Villarroel T, Clokie CM, Feine JS. Differences between sexes in postsurgical pain. Pain 2000;85:79–85.

20. Flood AB, Lorence DP, Ding G, McPherson K, Black NA. The role of expectations in patients' reports of post-operative outcomes and improvement following therapy. Med Care 1993;31:1043–1056.

21. Lick J, Bootzin R. Expectancy factors in the treatment of fear: Methodological and theoretical issues. Psychol Bull 1975;82:917.

22. Allen FP, McMillan AS, Walshaw D. Patient expectations of oral implant-retained prostheses in a UK dental hospital. Br Dent J 1999;23:80–84.

CHAPTER 5

Implant Overdentures Versus Conventional Dentures

Jocelyne S. Feine and Guido Heydecke

People who have lost all of their teeth suffer from a chronic condition. By definition, all treatment of a chronic condition is palliative, as there cannot be a *restitutio ad integrum*. Consequently, a patient has to live with all impacts on his or her well-being, those stemming from both the disease and the therapy. In the case of complete edentulism, impacts of disease are the obvious disfigurement, impaired speech, and problems with biting and chewing.

Traditional prosthetic rehabilitation of edentulous patients focuses on the replacement of structure with removable prostheses. However, the "therapeutic" effect may not be complete; although improved, function still may be impaired with clinically acceptable dentures.

Traditionally, the condition of an edentulous patient has been measured in clinical terms, such as ridge height and profile or the position and quality of the mucosa.[1-3] The clinical success of complete denture treatment has been measured using bite force[4] and functional tests of chewing capacity and efficiency.[5,6] However, correlations between clinical measures and the condition reported by the patient are often poor and nonsignificant (Table 5-1). These poor correlations between clinical factors and

patient assessments emphasize that while prosthetic therapy in the past has focused on restoring lost structure, function, and esthetics, the edentulous condition affects patients on a personal level. Research only recently has shifted toward surveying edentulous patients regarding their priorities for complete denture treatment. For patients, the most important qualities of complete dentures are comfort, stability, and ability to chew with the denture. Other factors include esthetics, ability to speak, and ease of cleaning the denture.[7,8]

Satisfaction

Satisfaction as an outcome measure has experienced a renaissance in the past 10 years. Satisfaction describes the patient's valuation of a specific aspect of (denture) treatment. As with most patient outcomes, satisfaction is measured using self-administered questionnaires. Categories of measurement include general satisfaction, satisfaction with stability, comfort, esthetics, speech, chewing ability, and ease of cleaning. For scaling purposes, questions are either coupled with multi-step an-

Table 5-1 Correlations between clinical parameters and patient assessments in edentulous patients with conventional dentures

Clinical parameters	Patient parameters	Correlation	Reference
Anatomical factors			
Anatomical condition	Overall result	0.28	1
	General satisfaction	0.22	3
Bone height (radiographically determined)	General satisfaction	0.15	2
Assessment of ridge	General satisfaction	0.12	2
Soft tissue resilience, mobility	General satisfaction	0.06	3
Resorption of ridge	Chewing ability	0.33*	5
Technical factors			
Stability of prosthesis	Overall result	0.44	1
Retention of prosthesis	Overall result	0.12	1
Assessment of old prosthesis	General satisfaction	−0.22	3
Technical quality of prosthesis	General satisfaction	0.36*	2
Chewing capacity	Chewing ability	0.34*	5
General ratings			
Overall result	Overall result	0.8*	1
Assessment of problem	General satisfaction	0.31*	3
Overall clinical assessment	General satisfaction	0.12	2

*Statistically significant.

swer categories (Likert scales) or visual analog scales (VAS; Fig 5-1).

Dissatisfaction with complete denture treatment among edentulous patients has been an issue for many years. For instance, a survey of elderly patients showed 66% were dissatisfied with their complete dentures. The main reasons for dissatisfaction were discomfort, poor fit and retention, and especially soreness and pain under mandibular dentures, which can cause many more problems than maxillary dentures.[3,9]

It has been shown that the satisfaction with conventional dentures and implant overdentures depends on patients' ability to chew and speak and on the appearance of the prostheses.[1,10,11]

Carlsson et al[1] proposed that self-ratings of retention and the sense of security with the denture also contribute to patient satisfaction with complete dentures.

Several studies have compared simple mandibular overdentures supported by two implants to conventional complete dentures using a questionnaire approach. However, few studies are randomized controlled trials; only these will be reviewed here.

Researchers from the Netherlands conducted a randomized multicenter study (90 patients) to compare patient satisfaction with mandibular conventional dentures (n = 30), with conventional dentures combined with surgical vestibuloplasty (n = 30), and with over-

"Are you satisfied with the comfort of your mandibular prosthesis?"

Not at all   Extremely
satisfied   satisfied

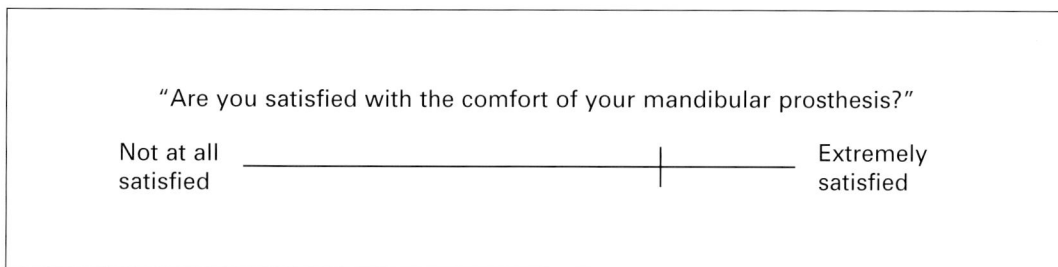

Fig 5-1 Example of a visual analog scale (VAS) question with the patient's response as a vertical line across the horizontal line.

dentures supported by two implants (n = 30). A validated questionnaire (test-retest reliability r = 0.8 to 0.9) targeted patient satisfaction with esthetics, retention, functional comfort, and the ability to eat and speak with the dentures, all rated on 5-point scales. General satisfaction was rated on a 10-point scale. One year posttreatment, general satisfaction with implant overdentures and conventional dentures combined with vestibuloplasty was significantly higher than with conventional dentures alone. No significance tests were reported for the other parameters.[12,13] Five years posttreatment, the positive effect of vestibuloplasty had disappeared and the difference with conventional treatment alone was no longer significant. However, implant overdentures consistently produced significantly higher general satisfaction scores compared to both alternative treatments.[14]

Similar results were reported by Geertman et al.[15,16] In a randomized trial of 151 patients, 60 received conventional complete dentures. Ninety-one patients had three different types of implants (transmandibular, hollow cylinder, and screw type) placed and were finally restored with mandibular implant overdentures retained by a bar-clip. Patients with implant overdentures had higher general satisfaction

ratings than patients with conventional dentures. No statistical comparisons were reported.[15,16]

In a randomized trial by Kapur et al,[17] new maxillary and mandibular dentures were delivered to diabetic denture patients who treated their diabetes either with or without insulin. Of 89 patients, 37 received maxillary and mandibular conventional dentures and 52 received a maxillary conventional denture and a mandibular implant overdenture. Questionnaires with categorical responses were used to ascertain patients' absolute assessments of original dentures at baseline and study dentures at 6 and 24 months after completion of treatment. While longitudinal data for the satisfaction questionnaire showed improvements with both types of study dentures, improvements were higher in the implant overdenture group than in the conventional denture group. Statistical evaluation of percentage distributions for the evaluation of the study dentures showed significant improvements in the implant overdenture group for eating enjoyment and general satisfaction. A significant between-group difference was detected for speech in favor of the implant overdenture group. Mean scores failed to show any significant differences between the two treatment groups. With the

Table 5-2 Mean scores (mm VAS) of posttreatment satisfaction ratings by adults aged 35 to 65 years

Variable	Conventional denture group	Overdenture group
	Mean (SD)	Mean (SD)
General satisfaction	63.7 (34.7)	89.2 (21.8)*
Comfort	63.6 (36.8)	88.9 (21.4)[†]
Esthetics	88.9 (17.8)	90.6 (14.9)
Ability to speak	85.2 (20.9)	91.7 (11.8)
Stability	64.5 (36.4)	90.6 (19.8)[†]
Ability to clean	89.9 (17.8)	91.1 (18.3)

*Significant between-group difference; t tests. $P \leq .001$.
[†]Significant between-group difference; t tests. $P < .05$.
Data from Awad et al.[18]

comparative questionnaire, a higher percentage of patients in the implant overdenture group than in the conventional denture group perceived improvements with study dentures from their original dentures in chewing ability, chewing comfort, and denture security.[17]

The authors have conducted several trials comparing mandibular conventional dentures and overdentures retained by two implants. In one of them, edentulous adults, aged 35 to 65 years, were randomly assigned to two groups that received either a mandibular conventional denture (n = 48) or an overdenture supported by two endosseous implants with a bar attachment (n = 54). Using VAS, patients rated their general satisfaction and other features of their original dentures and their new prostheses prior to treatment and 2 months after delivery.[18] The mean posttreatment general satisfaction was significantly higher in the overdenture group than in the conventional denture group. Further between-group differ-

ences were found for comfort and stability in favor of the implant overdenture (Table 5-2). Within the implant group, ratings had improved significantly for four additional aspects of the prostheses (comfort, esthetics, stability, and ease of chewing; $P < .05$). The authors concluded that a mandibular two-implant overdenture opposed by a maxillary conventional denture is a more effective treatment for edentulous middle-aged adults than conventional dentures on both arches.[18]

In a second study, 60 elderly edentulous patients (aged 65 to 75 years) were randomly assigned to receive a maxillary conventional denture along with either a mandibular conventional denture (n = 30) or a two-implant overdenture with ball retainers (n = 30). Prior to treatment and 2 and 6 months after delivery, patients rated their general satisfaction with their prostheses, as well as other features of their dentures using VAS. Patients who received the implant-supported overdentures rated their general satisfaction with the prostheses significantly higher than the conventional denture group (*P* < .01). In addition, the implant group gave significantly higher ratings to several other aspects of the prostheses (comfort, stability, ability to chew, and esthetics; *P* < .05). These results suggest that 2 and 6 months posttreatment, mandibular two-implant overdentures with maxillary conventional dentures provide significantly greater satisfaction than conventional dentures.[19]

Oral Health–Related Quality of Life

Middle-aged Adults

Bouma et al[20] reported that for 1-year posttreatment, all 32 patients (mean age 57.0, SD 12) who received mandibular two-implant overdentures with a bar attachment and those in the conventional denture group (n = 29, mean age 55.0, SD 11) had significant improvements on the Groningen Activity Restriction Scale-Dentistry (GARS-D), which measures the impact of prostheses on activities such as going out and contact with people. However, no between-group differences were observed. This led to questions about findings from other nonrandomized studies for which treatment differences were reported. However, up to 43% of patients in their trial had pretreatment scores of 0 on the GARS-D, indicating "no problems." Therefore, it is likely that this scale may not have been sensitive enough to detect between-group differences in oral health–related quality of life (QOL).[20]

Awad and coworkers[11] used the Oral Health Impact Profile (OHIP) to compare mandibular conventional dentures and overdentures retained by two implants in a group of 102 edentulous adults (aged 35 to 65 years). The origi-

nal OHIP is a 49-item profile that describes the impacts of oral health conditions on aspects of function, daily living, and social interactions in seven domains, including functional limitation, physical pain, psychological discomfort, physical disability, psychological disability, social disability, and handicap.[21] Items of the OHIP were scored on six-point scales (never, rarely, occasionally, often, very often, all the time), which were assigned numerical values between 1 (never) and 6 (all the time). Subscale and total scores were calculated by adding the item scores.

Patients were assigned randomly to two groups that received either a mandibular conventional denture (n = 48) or an overdenture supported by two endosseous implants with a bar-clip attachment (n = 54). Prior to and 2 months posttreatment, patients completed the 49-item OHIP. The implant overdenture group had a significantly better oral health–related QOL than the conventional denture group 2 months posttreatment. This was expressed in significantly lower scores in all OHIP domains. Total OHIP-49 scores also were significantly lower in the implant overdenture group. Compared to patients with implant overdentures, edentulous patients with conventional dentures have their QOL significantly impacted due to their condition.[11]

Older Adults

Similar findings were reported for a group of 60 elderly patients, who received either mandibular implant overdentures (n = 30) or conventional dentures (n = 30). Patients completed a 20-item short version of the Oral Health Impact Profile (OHIP-20) prior to treatment, then at 2 and 6 months after delivery of the dentures.[19,22]

Patients with implant overdentures had significantly fewer oral health–related QOL impacts than the conventional denture group.

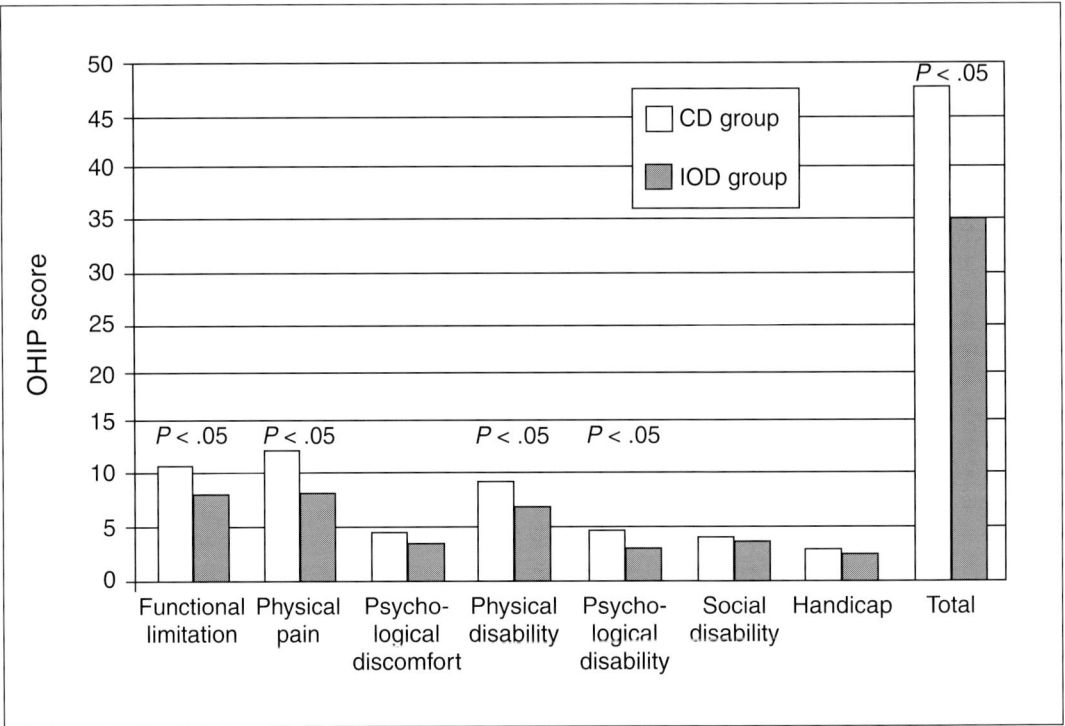

Fig 5-2 Six-month posttreatment OHIP-20 scores for each domain and the total score. The study population, aged 65 to 75 years, received either conventional dentures (CD) or implant overdentures (IOD). Significantly lower impact was found in the implant overdenture group (see *P* values). (Data from Heydecke et al.[22])

This was reflected in lower scores on three of the seven domains of the OHIP-20, namely functional limitation, physical pain, and physical disability, as well as on total OHIP-20 scores (*P* < .05).[19] Six months after delivery of the prostheses, OHIP-20 measurements were repeated. In addition to the 2-month follow-up, a fourth domain, psychological disability, reached significance (*P* < .05; Fig 5-2). Pre-posttreatment comparisons for implant patients yielded significant improvement on all subscales.

In conclusion, mandibular overdentures retained by two implants provide elderly patients with better oral health–related QOL.[22]

Function

In the Netherlands, 151 patients with severely resorbed mandibles participated in a multicenter randomized trial. Ninety-one patients received implant-retained mandibular overdentures and 60 patients received a conventional complete denture. Patients' experiences were evaluated before treatment and 1-year after insertion of the new dentures. Results before treatment showed that both treatment groups were comparable: They both were dissatisfied with their mandibular denture and they both could hardly chew tough or hard foods. One year posttreatment, patients in the implant overdenture group rated their ability to chew hard and tough foods significantly better than did the conventional denture group ($P < .0001$).[15,16]

Data from a further randomized trial in which 38 men and 52 women were assigned to three treatment modalities (conventional denture, n = 30; conventional denture with surgical vestibuloplasty, n = 30; and implant overdenture, n = 30) were evaluated by Boerrigter et al.[13] The outcome measures were functional complaints and chewing ability, assessed using questionnaires focused on denture-related complaints and the ability to chew different types of food. At the 1-year evaluation, five of seven factors showed significantly better scores for the implant overdenture and conventional denture/vestibuloplasty groups than for the control group (conventional denture only). For the scale-functional complaints with the mandibular denture, the implant overdenture group showed a significantly better score than the conventional denture/vestibuloplasty and the conventional denture–only groups. The ability to chew hard and tough foods was significantly better for the implant overdenture and conventional denture/vestibuloplasty groups than for conventional denture–only patients.[13]

In a randomized trial of 102 edentulous diabetic patients by Garrett et al,[23] treatment was completed in 89 patients, of which 37 received conventional dentures and 52 received implant overdentures with a bar-clip attachment supported by two implants. Masticatory tests were performed by patients before treatment and at 6 and 24 months posttreatment. For 68 patients (25 conventional denture, 43 implant overdenture) chewing performance data were available for both baseline and 6-month posttreatment sessions. All pretreatment masticatory performance scores with original dentures were higher in the conventional denture group than in the implant overdenture group. The posttreatment performance scores for the two treatment groups were similar because of the higher gains of the overdenture group. Due to the unequal pretreatment scores, implant overdentures showed no significant advantage over conventional dentures for improving the ability to comminute food in this group of diabetic patients.[23]

Self-reported functional data also were collected in a randomized trial by Awad et al.[18] Patients received either a mandibular conventional denture (n = 48) or an implant overdenture with a bar attachment (n = 54). Using VAS, anchored by the words "not at all difficult" to "impossible to chew," patients rated their general chewing ability and their ability to chew six different types of food (soft bread, hard cheese, dry sausage, lettuce, raw apple, and carrot) prior to and 2 and 6 months posttreatment. These foods were chosen from a list ranked in order of masticatory difficulty by patients with complete dentures.[10] The general ability to chew as well as to chew all types of foods was significantly higher for the implant group at 2 and 6 months (t tests, $P < .05$; Fig 5-3).[18]

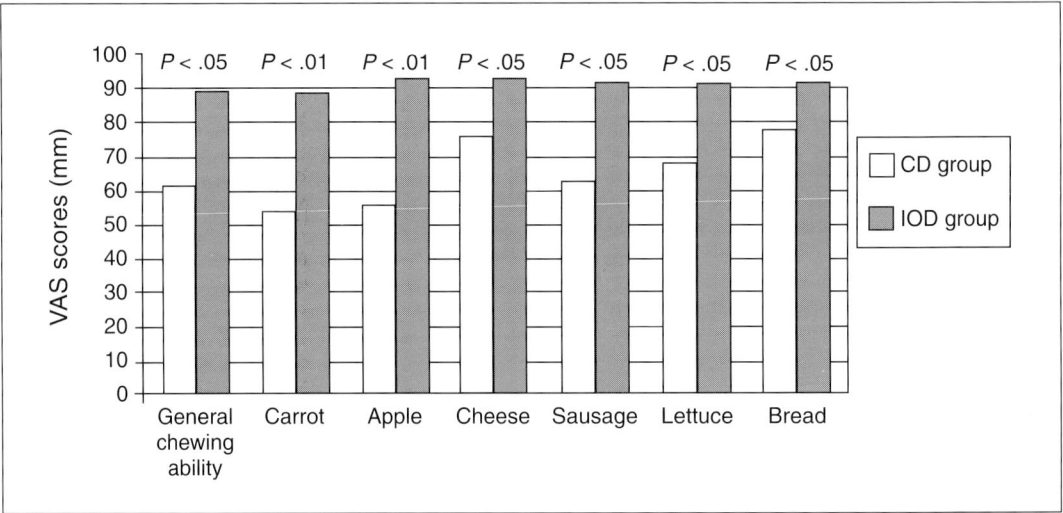

Fig 5-3 Patients' ratings of ability to chew different types of food. Patients with implant overdentures (IOD) rated their overall ability to chew significantly better than did patients with conventional dentures (CD). (Modified with permission from Awad et al.[18])

Conclusion

The data from the randomized trials reviewed in this chapter confirm that implant overdentures provide patients with better outcomes than do conventional dentures. These positive outcomes include psychosocial outcomes such as satisfaction and oral health–related quality of life, as well as functional outcomes such as chewing ability. This improved function with implant overdentures could increase the range of foods consumed by edentulous patients, which, in turn, also may improve their nutritional status and general health (see chapter 2).

Acknowledgments

The authors want to thank contributing author Manal Awad, BDS, PhD, Department of Mathematics and Statistics and Department of Health Services Administration, American University of Sharjah, Faculty of Health Sciences, United Arab Emirates.

This work was funded by University Industry grant No. UCT36052 from the Canadian Institutes of Health Research and Straumann Canada Limited.

References

1. Carlsson GE, Otterland A, Wennstrom A. Patient factors in appreciation of complete dentures. J Prosthet Dent 1967;17:322–328.
2. van Waas MA. The influence of clinical variables on patients' satisfaction with complete dentures. J Prosthet Dent 1990;63:307–310.
3. Berg E. The influence of some anamnestic, demographic, and clinical variables on patient acceptance of new complete dentures. Acta Odontol Scand 1984;42:119–127.
4. Lindquist LW, Carlsson GE, Hedegard B. Changes in bite force and chewing efficiency after denture treatment in edentulous patients with denture adaptation difficulties. J Oral Rehabil 1986;13:21–29.

5. Slagter AP, Olthoff LW, Bosman F, Steen WH. Masticatory ability, denture quality, and oral conditions in edentulous subjects. J Prosthet Dent 1992;68:299–307.

6. Wayler AH, Chauncey HH. Impact of complete dentures and impaired natural dentition on masticatory performance and food choice in healthy aging men. J Prosthet Dent 1983;49:427–433.

7. Kent G. Effects of osseointegrated implants on psychological and social well-being: A literature review. J Prosthet Dent 1992;68:515–518.

8. Awad MA, Feine JS. Measuring patient satisfaction with mandibular prostheses. Community Dent Oral Epidemiol 1998;26:400–405.

9. Pietrokovski J, Harfin J, Mostavoy R, Levy F. Oral findings in elderly nursing home residents in selected countries: Quality of and satisfaction with complete dentures. J Prosthet Dent 1995;73:132–135.

10. Bergman B, Carlsson GE. Review of 54 complete denture wearers. Patients' opinions 1 year after treatment. Acta Odontol Scand 1972;30:399–414.

11. Awad MA, Locker D, Korner-Bitensky N, Feine JS. Measuring the effect of intra-oral implant rehabilitation on health-related quality of life in a randomized controlled clinical trial. J Dent Res 2000;79:1659–1663.

12. Boerrigter EM, Geertman ME, Van Oort RP, et al. Patient satisfaction with implant-retained mandibular overdentures. A comparison with new complete dentures not retained by implants—a multicentre randomized clinical trial. Br J Oral Maxillofac Surg 1995;33:282–288.

13. Boerrigter EM, Stegenga B, Raghoebar GM, Boering G. Patient satisfaction and chewing ability with implant-retained mandibular overdentures: A comparison with new complete dentures with or without preprosthetic surgery. J Oral Maxillofac Surg 1995;53:1167–1173.

14. Raghoebar GM, Meijer HJ, Stegenga B, van't Hof MA, van Oort RP, Vissink A. Effectiveness of three treatment modalities for the edentulous mandible. A five-year randomized clinical trial. Clin Oral Implants Res 2000;11:195–201.

15. Geertman ME, Boerrigter EM, van't Hof MA, et al. Two-center clinical trial of implant-retained mandibular overdentures versus complete dentures—chewing ability. Community Dent Oral Epidemiol 1996;24:79–84.

16. Geertman ME, van Waas MA, van't Hof MA, Kalk W. Denture satisfaction in a comparative study of implant-retained mandibular overdentures: A randomized clinical trial. Int J Oral Maxillofac Implants 1996;11:194–200.

17. Kapur KK, Garrett NR, Hamada MO, et al. Randomized clinical trial comparing the efficacy of mandibular implant-supported overdentures and conventional dentures in diabetic patients. Part III: Comparisons of patient satisfaction. J Prosthet Dent 1999;82:416–427.

18. Awad MA, Lund JP, Dufresne E, Feine JS. Comparing the efficacy of mandibular implant-retained overdentures and conventional dentures among middle-aged edentulous patients: Satisfaction and functional assessment. Int J Prosthodont 2003;16:117–122.

19. Awad MA, Lund LP, Shapiro SH, et al. Oral health status and treatment satisfaction with mandibular implant overdentures and conventional dentures. A randomized trial in a senior population. Int J Prosthodont 2003 (in press).

20. Bouma J, Boerrigter LM, Van Oort RP, van Sonderen E, Boering G. Psychosocial effects of implant-retained overdentures. Int J Oral Maxillofac Implants 1997;12:515–522.

21. Slade GD, Spencer AJ. Development and evaluation of the oral health impact profile. Community Dent Health 1994;11:3–11.

22. Heydecke G, Locker D, Awad MA, Lund JP, Feine JS. Oral and general health status six months after treatment with mandibular implant overdentures and conventional dentures. A randomized trial in an elderly population. Community Dent Oral Epidemiol 2003 (in press).

23. Garrett NR, Kapur KK, Hamada MO, et al. A randomized clinical trial comparing the efficacy of mandibular implant-supported overdentures and conventional dentures in diabetic patients. Part II. Comparisons of masticatory performance. J Prosthet Dent 1998;79:632-640.

CHAPTER 6

Measuring the Cost of Implant Overdenture Therapy

John R. Penrod and Yoshiaki Takanashi

Dental implant treatment is a safe, efficacious, and effective therapy for edentulous arches.[1,2] However, the relatively high initial costs for current implant treatments often lead patients, especially the elderly, to choose the less expensive option—treatment with conventional dentures. This choice is driven in large part by patients' limited ability to pay; edentulous patients tend to come from households with below-average incomes.[3] Therefore, before implant therapy can become the standard of treatment for edentulous patients, cost-effective, simpler implant treatments that are affordable for patients must be developed. Economic data for such treatments would provide important information to all relevant parties: patients, health care providers, and third-party payers.

This chapter compares the cost of mandibular overdentures supported by two implants to conventional denture treatment through 1 year after delivery of the prosthesis. Because of their simplicity, mandibular overdentures supported by two implants with ball attachments may be less expensive than other implant treatments for which economic data are available.[4,5] This analysis was conducted alongside a randomized controlled trial involving 60 elderly edentulous patients in Montreal, Canada. A resource-based microcosting of the direct and indirect costs (in 1999 Canadian dollars) of all scheduled and unscheduled visits was conducted through 1 year after delivery of the prosthesis.

While implant overdentures are less expensive than implant-supported fixed prostheses, they do cost more than conventional dentures. The cost identification through year 1 is the first step in a long-term evaluation of the cost effectiveness of treatment modalities and, hence, a step toward the answer to the question, Are implant overdentures worth the cost?

Cost Analysis

The economic analysis was designed prospectively as part of a randomized controlled trial comparing the efficacy of overdentures supported by two implants to conventional dentures in patients aged 65 to 75 years. The primary outcome of the study was to assess the difference in patient satisfaction, and the primary endpoint was 2 months after delivery of the prosthesis. Patients who met all inclusion and exclusion criteria were asked to participate in the study.[6] Thirty patients in the implant overdenture group and 30 in the conventional denture group participated in the study. The overdenture patients received two root-form implants (ITI dental implant system, solid screw sandblasted, large-grit, acid-etched implants, Straumann, Waldenburg, Switzerland) placed in front of the mental foramina. Details of the clinical procedures have been described elsewhere.[6,7] To compare the two groups, Student t or Mann-Whitney U tests were performed with SPSS 10.0 (SPSS, Chicago, IL).

For the economic portion of the study, visits were subdivided into scheduled and unscheduled visits. Unscheduled visits were defined as visits initiated by patients.[6,7] The treatment was divided into one surgical phase and four prosthodontic phases, P1 to P4. The surgical phase was from preliminary examination to postoperative reline. P1 was from the day preliminary impressions were taken to the day of delivery; P2 was from the day of delivery to 2 months postdelivery; P3 was from 2 to 6 months postdelivery; and P4 was 6 months to 1 year postdelivery.

Cost Calculation

Costs were subdivided into direct and indirect costs and were estimated based on microcosting of the resources used (clinician time, etc), rather than clinician charges. The direct costs included costs of labor, materials, pharmaceuticals, laboratory work, and radiography. The indirect costs included patients' time and out-of-pocket expenses.

To determine the opportunity cost of labor, the time spent by the clinicians and the surgical assistant was measured. This time included setup, treatment, clean up, and administrative tasks associated with patient contact. A de-

tailed account of the time spent at each treatment stage has been reported previously.[6,7] The opportunity cost of time was estimated from data on Quebec incomes from the 1996 Canadian census.[8] Adjusted to 1999 dollars, the average hourly wages of dentists and dental assistants were Can $51.97 and Can $15.87, respectively. Since there are no data available on the incomes of Canadian oral surgeons, data on clinician incomes from the United States were used to calculate the ratio of specialist-to-generalist incomes. This ratio was applied to the 1996 Canadian census data to obtain an estimated value of an oral surgeon's time of Can $73/h.[9] Since the American Dental Association (ADA) data indicated that the wages of American prosthodontists and general practitioners are quite similar, the prosthodontist's wage was estimated at Can $52/h.[10] Costs of nonmonetary "fringe" benefits of clinicians and staff were included in the overhead costs described below.

All disposable and reusable materials used for both groups were recorded. A product catalog (Henry Schein Arcona, Canada) from 1999 was used for acquiring market prices of all materials. To estimate the cost per use of reusable items, 28 Montreal-area dentists were asked to fill out a questionnaire regarding the useful life and the frequency of use per week of the relevant items. Using the useful life, the purchase price, and a discount rate of 5%, the annualized costs were computed using the standard textbook calculation.[11] The cost per use then was estimated by dividing the equivalent annual cost by the frequency of usage in one year, provided by the clinician survey.

Laboratory costs were based on the fee of a commercial dental laboratory in Montreal and pharmaceutical prices were obtained from a Montreal retail pharmacy. Radiographs were covered by the Régie de l'assurance maladie du Québec, the universal provincial health care insurance plan. The cost for one panoramic radiograph, Can $27.23, was used for the cost calculation and was provided by the administrators of the Royal Victoria Hospital. The radiographs are read by the oral surgeon and the cost of radiograph evaluation is included in his time cost. Indirect costs included patients' time of seeking treatment and their transportation. Following the recommendations of published guidelines, the human capital method was used to value this time.[12,13] The average of hourly earnings reported in the 1996 Canadian census for Quebec workers aged 55 and older, Can $17.16 (adjusted for inflation to 1999 Canadian dollars), was used. Transportation costs included hospital parking, taxis, public transportation, and patients' own motor vehicle operation. Estimates of transportation costs were based on a patient self-administered questionnaire.

Overhead costs

The cost analysis for this study reflects the costs of resources directly associated with treatment or, in the case of indirect costs, with seeking treatment. However, a significant portion of overall cost is related to the overhead of operation of the dental practice. As time required by prosthodontists is similar for both treatment modalities studied here, incorporation of overhead costs does not significantly impact the estimated cost *difference*. Nevertheless, adoption or nonadoption of an implant strategy is likely to influence the long-term number of oral surgery practices. For this reason, it is important to incorporate overhead practice expenses.

Although no published data on practice expenses in Canada are available, the ADA published estimates of overhead and other expenses as a percentage of the gross billing of solo unincorporated specialists practicing in the United States.[14] Adjusting the ADA data to accommodate the particular features of the practices studied in this chapter, the practice overhead was calculated to be 40% and 38% of total billings for oral surgeons and prosthodontists, respectively. Since the ADA data showed that gross billings were roughly two times specialist income, two times the estimated clinician expense was used as the base figure to apply the overhead rate.

Clinician Treatment Time

For the oral surgeon, the greatest time requirement was during the surgical phase, not surprisingly. Overall the oral surgeon spent an average of just under 2 hours with each patient in the overdenture group (113 minutes), with a mean of 106 minutes in the surgical phase, a mean of 6 minutes in P1, and a mean of 1 minute in P4. For the conventional denture group, the oral surgeon spent a mean of 5 minutes in P4.

Figure 6-1 shows the differences in the restorative dentist's time by stage. The restorative dentist required an average of 46 minutes during the surgical period; 29 of those minutes were for postoperative relines. The time required by the restorative dentist during the prosthodontic phases (P1 to P4) was quite similar for both the overdenture group (329 minutes) and the conventional denture group (337 minutes), and the difference was not statistically significant ($P = .47$). However, the combination of time required in the surgical and prosthodontic phases resulted in the restorative dentist having spent more time with the overdenture group than the conventional denture group, 376 minutes and 337 minutes, respectively ($P = .02$).

The total clinician time (for both the restorative dentist and the oral surgeon) was 489 minutes for the overdenture group and

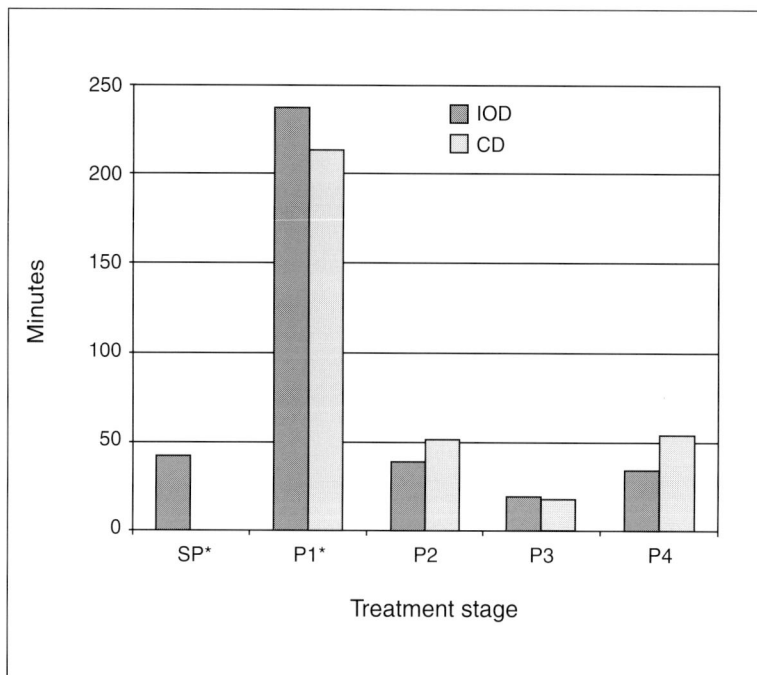

Fig 6-1 Mean time spent by the restorative dentist for each treatment stage. (IOD) Implant overdenture; (CD) complete denture; (SP) surgical phase; (P) prosthodontic phase. (*P < .05.)

342 minutes for the conventional denture group (P < .001). Again, the difference is entirely due to clinician time in the surgical phase. A detailed breakdown of clinician time by treatment period and by scheduled and unscheduled visits has been reported previously.[6,7]

Cost of Scheduled and Unscheduled Visits

Table 6-1 summarizes the total direct and indirect costs by treatment group. Again, direct costs were the opportunity cost of the clinicians' time plus the cost of materials and labo-

ratory fees. Indirect costs are the opportunity cost of patients' time and transportation.

The direct costs, including overhead of all treatment stages through 1-year follow-up, were Can $2,850 for the overdenture group and Can $1,193 for the conventional denture group. The difference in total direct costs between the two groups was statistically significant (Student t test; P < .001). The overdenture–conventional denture direct cost ratio was 1:2.4.

Although the difference in overall direct costs was substantial, this difference was due to treatment costs during the period up to delivery. Examination of direct costs during the fol-

Table 6-1 Mean (SD) of direct and indirect costs (in 1999 Canadian dollars) for scheduled and unscheduled visits (n = 30)

	Overdenture group*	Conventional denture group*
Direct cost less overhead cost	2,490 (278)	962 (272)
Direct cost including overhead cost	2,850 (330)	1,193 (371)
Indirect cost	1,395 (252)	1,123 (416)
Total cost less overhead cost	3,885 (504)	2,085 (675)
Total cost including overhead cost	4,245 (565)	2,316 (774)

*All differences between the groups are statistically significant at $P < .05$ (Student t test).

low-up periods (P2 to P4) revealed that the unconditional median (interquartile range, IQR) direct costs in the overdenture group and the conventional denture group did not differ much (Can $113, SD 138, and Can $92, SD 154, respectively).

Indirect costs over the course of the study for both the overdenture and conventional denture groups were quite similar, Can $1,395 and Can $1,123, respectively (see Table 6-1), though this difference in cost was found to be statistically significant (Student t test; $P = .003$). For the follow-up periods (P2 to P4), IQR indirect costs from P2 to P4 were Can $314 (SD 227) in the overdenture group and $386 (SD 341) in the conventional denture group; there was no statistical difference ($P = .212$).

For the combination of both direct and indirect costs, the mean total costs over the course of the study were Can $4,245 for the overdenture group and Can $2,316 for the conventional denture group (see Table 6-1), a statistically significant difference ($P < .001$). Including direct and indirect costs, the overdenture–conventional denture cost ratio was 1:1.8.

Long-term Implications of Cost Analysis

The cost comparison is important because the implant modality evaluated in this chapter is simpler and potentially less costly than previously evaluated implant prostheses. In contrast to most published studies of implant-supported prostheses versus conventional dentures, cost estimates for this study were based on observed resource utilization and the opportunity costs of these resources rather than solely on clinician fees. Health economists and various government bodies charged with health technology assessment have described the ways in which fee data may be inappropriate for use in economic analysis.[12,13,15] In addition, this study incorporates patients' time and transportation costs. Published guidelines for health technology assessment recommend a social perspective whereby this burden on patients is incorporated.[12,13] The study discussed in this chapter was the first study of prosthesis provision to include patients' indirect costs.

Since the overdenture–conventional denture cost ratio (using only direct costs) has been reported in previous work, we also calculated this ratio as part of our study. This statistic allows for comparison of the cost of the various implant therapies in various countries against a common standard—the cost of conventional denture treatment. In this study, the total direct costs for the overdenture group (Can $2,850) were 2.4 times more than the costs for the conventional denture group (Can $1,193), for all scheduled and unscheduled visits up to 1 year postdelivery. The two main determinants of this difference were *(1)* the cost of the implant and ball attachment materials and *(2)* the clinician's time associated with the surgical stage of implant treatment. Although mandibular overdentures supported by two implants exhibited complications in previous studies,[16] for the overdentures examined here, no between-group difference in the cost of unscheduled visits through 1 year postdelivery was observed.

The indirect patient costs of implant provision are substantial; through 1 year postdelivery, these costs were Can $1,395 for the overdenture group and $1,123 for the conventional denture group. Although the difference in indirect costs is statistically significant, the overall indirect patient burden appears similar. The indirect cost difference corresponds to the three additional visits required by the overdenture group (17.5 versus 14.2 visits).

A previous paper assessed the cost of implant-supported fixed prostheses, estimating that implant treatment costs are 6.5 times greater than those of conventional denture treatment.[4] Although that study had a longer follow-up period (5 years), the difference from the ratio calculated in this chapter can be explained largely by the differences in implant prostheses studied. The implant-supported fixed prosthesis evaluated in the previous study[4] required multiple implants and surgery in multiple stages, whereas the implant modality studied here required only one surgery.

An earlier Canadian study examined the costs of ball attachment implant prostheses.[17] However, it focused only on the fabrication period (P1) and relied on clinician fees in British Columbia rather than on a microcosting of the time and materials required for fabrication. The mean cost of fabrication of a three-implant prosthesis with ball attachments was reported to be Can $2,363, excluding the surgical procedures.[17] The estimated cost for the corresponding treatment period in this study was Can $1,428. Because the time and material resources used by the British Columbia clinicians were not reported, it is impossible to determine whether the differences are due to differences in resources utilized, interprovincial differences in the cost of these resources, or a deviation of British Columbia clinician fees from true economic costs.

One recent study compared the cost of mandibular overdentures supported by two implants to conventional denture treatment using the microcosting method, excluding patient indirect costs.[5] The surgical phase for the implant modality evaluated in that study used different techniques from the one studied in this chapter; however, a similar amount of clinician time required during the prosthodontic phase was found in the study noted in this chapter. The result from the previous study, that mandibular overdentures supported by two implants with a single-bar attachment cost 3.08 times more than conventional dentures in the first year, is similar to, though higher than, our estimate of 2.4. The difference can be explained largely by the fact that the implant system in the previous study required two surgical visits, confirming our hypothesis that the simpler implant modality evaluated in this study is less resource intensive and, therefore, less costly than previously evaluated implant modalities.

The study reviewed in this chapter has several limitations. First, the data are from one clinician of each type. Second, the study was conducted in a teaching hospital with specialists. Although care was taken to define the treatment protocol as similar to the general practice setting as possible (Awad et al, unpublished data, 2002), it is possible that the care provided by the clinicians in our study could be different from that provided in general practices. Finally, long-term data on both effectiveness and costs are required for a complete economic evaluation. These data will be studied as they become available. The long-term cost-effectiveness analysis will help the relevant parties—patients, clinicians, and third-party payers—determine whether implant overdentures are worth the cost.

Given the high costs for dental implant treatment and the relatively low incomes of the edentulous population, simpler treatments and related costs and effectiveness must be studied before implant treatment becomes the standard of care for edentulous patients. For the cost-effectiveness calculation, the cost and effectiveness data must be long term, which in this case, means the remaining life of the patients. Although the authors will continue to collect both cost and effectiveness data, modeling of profiles of costs and effectiveness for the very long term will be required. The modeling exercise will be based on published data and expert opinion.

Acknowledgment

This study was supported by a University Industry Partnership Grant from the Canadian Institutes of Health Reseach and Straumann Canada Limited.

References

1. Adell R, Eriksson B, Lekholm U, Brånemark PI, Jemt T. Long-term follow-up study of osseointegrated implants in the treatment of totally edentulous jaws. Int J Oral Maxillofac Implants 1990;5:347–359.
2. Lindquist LW, Carlsson GE, Jemt T. A prospective 15-year follow-up study of mandibular fixed prostheses supported by osseointegrated implants. Clinical results and marginal bone loss. Clin Oral Implants Res 1996;7:329–336 [erratum 1997;8:342].
3. Oral Health in America: A Report of the Surgeon General. Rockville, MD: US Department of Health and Human Services, National Institute of Dental and Craniofacial Research, National Institutes of Health, 2000.
4. Jönsson B, Karlsson G. Cost-benefit evaluation of dental implants. Int J Technol Assess Health Care 1990;6:545–557.
5. van der Wijk P, Bouma J, van Waas MA, van Oort RP, Rutten FF. The cost of dental implants as compared to that of conventional strategies. Int J Oral Maxillofac Implants 1998;13:546–553.
6. Takanashi Y, Penrod JR, Chehade A, et al. Does a prosthodontist spend more time providing mandibular 2-implant overdentures than conventional dentures? Int J Prosthodont 2002;15:397–403.
7. Takanashi Y, Penrod JR, Chehade A, Klemetti E, Lund JP, Feine JS. Surgical placement of two implants in the anterior edentulous mandible: How much time does it take? Clin Oral Implants Res 2003 (in press).
8. 1996 Census of Canada. The 1996 dimension series. Selected labour force, demographic, cultural, educational and income characteristics by sex, showing detailed occupation, for Canada, provinces, territories and census metropolitan areas: Quebec, Catalogue no. 94F0009XDB96123. Ottawa, Canada: Ministry of Supply and Service, 2001.
9. The 1998 Survey of Dental Practice: Oral and Maxillofacial Surgeons in Private Practice. Chicago: American Dental Association, 1998.
10. The 1999 Survey of Dental Practice: Prosthodontists in Private Practice. Chicago: American Dental Association, 1999.
11. Drummond MF, O'Brien BJ, Stoddart GL, Torrance GW. Methods for the economic evaluation of medical care programmes, ed 2. New York: Oxford University Press, 1997.

12. Gold MR, Siegel JE, Russell LB, Weinstein MC (eds). Cost-effectiveness in Health and Medicine. Oxford: Oxford University Press, 1996.

13. Canadian Coordinating Office for Health Technology Assessment. Guidelines for Economic Evaluation of Pharmaceuticals: Canada, ed 2. Ottawa, Canada: Canadian Coordinating Office for Health Technology Assessment, 1997.

14. The 2000 Survey of Dental Practice: Annual Expenses of Operating a Private Practice. Chicago: American Dental Association, 2000.

15. Finkler SA. The distinction between cost and charges. Ann Intern Med 1982;96:102–109.

16. Naert I, Gizani S, Vuylsteke M, van Steenberghe D. A 5-year prospective randomized clinical trial on the influence of splinted and unsplinted oral implants retaining a mandibular overdenture: Prosthetic aspects and patient satisfaction. J Oral Rehabil 1999;26: 195–202.

17. Walton JN, MacEntee MI, Hanvelt R. Cost analysis of fabricating implant prostheses. Int J Prosthodont 1996;9:271–276.

CHAPTER 7

Choosing an Implant System for Clinical Practice: An Evidence-Based Method

Timothy W. Head

More than 50 companies manufacture "root-form" dental implants based on the principle of osseointegration. Many of these companies manufacture more than one implant design. This situation presents clinicians with a somewhat daunting task when deciding which implant system will be best for their patients. The experienced clinician likely will have developed confidence in the performance of the implant system or systems used in his or her practice. However, manufacturers will continually present new claims of improved performance, ease-of-use, and cost effectiveness. Those clinicians just beginning to employ implant dentistry in their practice lack the clinical experience on which to base their decisions, and therefore face a greater challenge. Both experienced and inexperienced clinicians should develop a strategy to select the most appropriate implant system for their patients. A reasonable starting point for this strategy is confirmation that the appropriate government authority has licensed the implant system under consideration. A second point of reference is verification that the appropriate national dental association has approved the implant system. Third, and most important, the

clinician should determine if the system can be validated by publications in peer-reviewed literature. This chapter reviews the application of this validation strategy in the United States and Canada.

Government Agencies

In the United States, the Food and Drug Administration (FDA) is responsible for monitoring the safety and effectiveness of medical devices. The distribution of dental implants is controlled by this agency. The FDA's objective is not to be a testing facility, but instead is to determine that data and results supplied by private sources follow FDA program guidelines. At one point, dental implants were placed in the Class III medical devices category, which required premarket approval. Premarket approval is a demanding process that includes controlled preclinical and clinical studies documenting an implant system's efficacy before it is allowed to enter the commercial market. No dental implant manufacturer has completed the premarket approval process. Manufacturers have been able to market their products by demonstrating "substantial equivalence" to previously approved devices. This form of approval is known as 510(k) or *premarket notification*. Devices do not have to be identical to previously marketed implants to be classified as substantially equivalent. The manufacturer is required to demonstrate only the same intended use (such as for edentulous, partially edentulous, or single-tooth applications) and the same technological characteristics. Manufacturers must provide a detailed narrative of the design characteristics, including diagrams, material specifications, and tolerances; sterilization information and labeling details; and results of static and fatigue testing in compression and shear. If the implant has the same intended use, but with different technological characteristics, then safety and effectiveness must be demonstrated. Corrosion tests and toxicology tests are required only when a new material is used that has not been identified in a previously marketed device. Animal and/or clinical studies are required only for implants with a diameter of less than 3 mm and lengths shorter than 7 mm and for abutments with angulations greater than 30 degrees.[1,2] Clinical data is not needed for most devices cleared by 510(k).[3]

Organized Dentistry

The American Dental Association (ADA) has, as part of its Seal of Acceptance program, an acceptance program for endosseous implants. This is a voluntary program for which a manufacturer must supply evidence of physical properties (eg, modulus of elasticity, strength, and hardness); tests establishing biocompatibility; and clinical studies including two independent prospective clinical studies with a minimum success rate of 85% and in which 60% of the cases were single-tooth or short-span fixed partial denture restorations. Provisional accep-

tance is awarded when 3-year follow-up clinical studies have been completed, and full acceptance is awarded when the clinical studies include a 5-year follow-up. Interested readers can visit the ADA's website for an update of the implant systems that have received the ADA Seal of Acceptance.[4]

Peer-Reviewed Literature Analysis

A paper by Eckert et al[5] underlines the clinical importance of reviewing the scientific literature concerning a particular implant system prior to its use in clinical practice. In 1991 Eckert and colleagues contacted six dental implant manufacturers and requested references to scientific articles that could validate the manufacturers' implant systems. These companies were selected because they had received provisional or full certification from the ADA or because they maintained a significant share of the North American dental implant market at that time. Each article was reviewed to determine whether it validated the particular implant system. Validation was based on criteria that were considered to be the minimum needed to describe the study as a "scientific study." The studies had to follow the standard format with introduction, methods and materials, results, analysis, and discussion. Articles were designated as *prospective* or *retrospective* studies if they fulfilled the criteria described for a "scientific study" and could validate the design in question. Conversely, unproved or untested hypotheses, clinical reports, literature reviews, and prospective or retrospective studies that lacked data collection and analysis were not considered to be validating articles. In addition, Eckert and colleagues identified the number of validating articles that described human (clinical) trials. They then repeated this process in

Table 7-1 Review of literature supplied by implant manufacturers

Manufacturer/ Implant system	1991 study			1995 study		
	No. of references submitted	Validating studies	Human studies	No. of references submitted	Validating articles	Strong validation
Calcitek						
Integral	10	5	0	15	6	0
Dentsply						
Core-Vent	19	0	0	0	0	0
Interpore						
IMZ	23	5	3	19	4	1
Noble Biocare						
Brånemark	5	5	5	13	12	8
Steri-Oss	14	0	0	0	0	0
Straumann						
ITI	12	6	3	11	4	0

Data modified from Eckert et al.[5]

1995, and in addition to determining the number of validating articles submitted by each manufacturer, they assigned a category of "strong" validation if the article provided evidence of research that demonstrated (1) objective success criteria, (2) data analysis, and (3) documentation of at least 5 years of clinical performance. A summary of the findings of these two literature reviews can be seen in Table 7-1.

Despite FDA and ADA approval of implant systems reviewed at the time of the literature review, clinicians cannot depend on these approval mechanisms alone and must accept some responsibility for reviewing the pertinent literature concerning an implant system.

The Canadian Dental Association has no mechanism for implant approval, although the Dental Materials and Devices Committee is considering this for the future. The sale of dental endosseous implants is regulated under the Medical Devices Regulations of the Food and Drug Act, administered by Health Canada. Dental implants are categorized as Class III devices, which must be approved in order to be imported into and sold in Canada. To receive approval, a manufacturer must submit a premarket review document. In brief, this document must include device description, design philosophy, marketing history, summary of safety and effectiveness, list of standards, method of sterilization, summary of studies (preclinical and clinical),

Table 7-2 Summary of findings from Medline search for peer-reviewed literature that could validate the implant systems approved by Health Canada

Manufacturer/ Implant system	No. of articles retrieved by Medline search	No. of validating clinical trials	No. of valid trials on overdentures
Ace Surgical Supply			
Ace Dental implant system	0	0	0
Basic Dental Implant System			
Basic dental implant	0	0	0
Bego			
Implant dentaire semados	1	0	0
Bicon			
Bicon dental implant	3	0	0
Biohorizons Implant Systems			
Maestro implant system	3	1	0
Core-Vent			
Paragon implant	18	1	0
Dentsply Friadent			
Frialit-2	30	2	0
Implant Innovations			
Osseotite	30	5	0
Self-tapping threaded implant	5	5	0
Cylinder implants	0	0	0
Imtec			
Imtec dental implants	3	0	0
Innova			
Endopore	11	5	2
Lifecore Biomedical			
Restore Close Tolerance Implant	1	0	0
Sustain dental implant system	0	0	0
Stage-1 single-stage dental implant	0	0	0
Nobel Biocare			
Brånemark	468	62	9
IMZ Interpore	103	12	8
Steri-Oss	22	3	0
Serf			
Implant Dentaire Evolution	1	0	0
Sterngold Implamed			
Endosseous dental implant	0	0	0
Straumann			
ITI dental implant system	170	34	11
Sulzer Calcitek			
Omnilock dental implant system	4	1	0
Spline dental implant system	9	0	0
Tenax Implant			
Tenax dental implant system	0	0	0

Criteria for Validating a Clinical Trial Article

- Appears in a peer-reviewed journal
- Contains introduction, methods and materials, results, analysis, and discussion
- Is a human trial
- Is prospective
- Contains objective success criteria
- Includes data analysis
- Has a minimum 3-year follow-up

and bibliography (all published reports).[6] Table 7-2 lists the 17 companies that have received Health Canada approval for their implant systems. This table also summarizes the findings of a search for peer-reviewed literature on implant systems, carried out using PubMed/Medline (www.ncbi.nlm.nih.gov/entrez/query) using the search strategy "dental implants AND implant company or implant system name." Companies for which no references were retrieved by this search were contacted and invited to submit relevant articles they felt validated their implant system(s). The references retrieved by this search were then reviewed to determine whether they met the criteria for valid clinical trials (see box).

For the purposes of this book, articles related to the use of implants for overdentures were identified as well. This preliminary literature review is limited in that it only identifies articles that appear to contain the components of a scientifically valid article. A more precise article review presently is being carried out following a protocol similar to that used by Eckert et al.[5] The relative scarcity of available articles for some implant systems should alert clinicians to the need to seek sufficient validation of an implant system prior to using it in clinical practice.

Summary

An appropriate strategy for selecting an implant system for general clinical use or for a specific clinical application should include: (1) verification that the system has approval by the appropriate government agency (Health Canada or the FDA); (2) verification that the appropriate national dental association (ADA or Canadian Dental Association) has approved the implant system in question, if that association has such an approval mechanism; and, most importantly, (3) a personal review of the validity of the literature made available by implant manufacturers and by searching databases such as Medline. It is only through this type of rigorous validation that the practice of evidence-based dentistry can be ensured and that patients can be provided with the most reliable implant systems available.

References

1. Eckert SE. Food and Drug Administration requirements for dental implants. J Prosthet Dent 1995;74:162–168.
2. Binon PP. Implants and components: Entering the new millennium. Int J Oral Maxillofac Implants 2000;15:76–94.
3. Premarket Notification 510(k): Regulatory Requirements for Medical Devices. Food and Drug Administration. Available at: www.fda.gov/cdrh/510khome.html. Accessed: May 2003.
4. The American Dental Association Website, Professional pages. Available at: www.ada.org/prof/prac/seal/sealsrch.asp. Accessed: May 2003.
5. Eckert SE, Parein A, Myshin HL, Padilla JL. Validation of dental implant systems through a review of literature supplied by system manufacturers. J Prosthet Dent 1997;77:271–279.
6. Preparation of a Premarket Review Document for Class III and Class IV Device License Applications. Available at: www.hc-sc.gc.ca/hpb_dgps/therapeut/htmleng/guidmd.html. Accessed: May 2003.

CHAPTER 8

Comparison of Treatment Strategies for Implant Overdentures

Daniel Wismeijer and Geert T. Stoker

Implants can be used to restore the edentulous mandible in different ways. For many patients, a fixed prosthesis can be placed on four or more dental implants, and long-term results for implant-retained fixed prostheses have been documented in the literature by various authors.[1–4] Implant-supported removable overdentures using two or more implants are also a possible treatment option for patients who have problems with conventional dentures.[5–14]

Overdentures obtain support and retention from a superstructure attached to the implants. This superstructure defines the character of the denture that can be created. One can differentiate between tissue-supported, tissue-implant–supported, and mainly implant-supported overdentures. In the tissue-supported overdenture on two implants, the retentive mechanism is a magnet or a ball attachment. The denture rests on the mucosal tissues and the attachments ensure retention only during lateral and extrusive movements.

A tissue-implant–supported overdenture provides retention via a superstructure on two implants interconnected by a bar attached to two gold caps that are screwed onto the implants. This denture rests on the mucosal tissues on the dorsal denture-bearing areas and on the bar and implants in the anterior regions; the bar is the axis over which the denture can rotate. Retention is ensured during lateral and extrusive forces. During "intrusive" forces, the implants carry the occlusal loading of the denture in the anterior region, but in the dorsal region of the denture-bearing area, the mucosal tissues are loaded.

An implant-supported overdenture placed on four implants rests primarily on the superstructure connected to the implants. In most situations, the superstructure is placed on four interconnected implants. During occlusal function the mucosal denture-bearing areas are minimally loaded.

There are several arguments in the literature to indicate a preference for one of the three treatment strategies. Challenges are discussed such as pain caused by denture pressure, the amount of available bone, the expected level of oral hygiene, patient expectations of the new appliance, and the maxillomandibular relationship, as well as therapy cost effectiveness.[10,14] While many studies have been published on implants and overdentures, only a few have compared the above-mentioned treatment options. The only study design that allows for a comparison of different types of treatment for patients with the same problem is a randomized controlled clinical trial.[15,16] Several randomized clinical trials on implant overdentures can be found in the literature.[17–26]

Treatment success is determined by more factors than the survival of the implants alone. An important factor in patient treatment is patient satisfaction. When there are multiple treatment options for edentulous patients, it is important to determine how the patient perceives the treatment and how satisfied he or she is after treatment. It also is important to consider the clinical performance of the entire treatment strategy. Next to peri-implant and radiographic parameters, problems concerning prosthetic maintenance must be taken into consideration. Another important consideration is the efficacy of the treatment. Evaluation of the total results of patient satisfaction, costs, and treatment aftercare provides insight into the total treatment result and can be compared for the three different treatment strategies.

This chapter describes the patient satisfaction, type and amount of prosthetic aftercare, and clinical performance associated with mandibular overdentures on dental implants. Overdentures on four interconnected implants are significantly more expensive to provide than are overdentures on two implants, and both types of denture are equally acceptable to patients. This means that mandibular overdentures on two implants is the more favorable option in implant overdenture treatment. Furthermore, the two-implant overdenture with bar retention is more cost-effective than the two-implant overdenture with ball retention, mostly because patients were more satisfied with the former while the long-term costs involved with the aftercare of both is about the same.

The Breda Implant Overdenture Study

The Breda Implant Overdenture Study (BIOS) was set up as a randomized controlled clinical trial to compare three different treatment options for edentulous patients using the ITI dental implant system (Straumann, Waldenburg, Switzerland). One hundred ten edentulous patients with atrophic mandibles and persistent conventional complete denture problems who were referred by their dentist to the Department of Oral and Maxillofacial Surgery and/or the Department of Special Dental Care and Maxillofacial Prosthodontics of the Ignatius Teaching Hospital, in Breda, The Netherlands, during the years 1991 to 1993 were treated with one-stage ITI dental implants and implant-retained overdentures. During the consultation, the medical status and dental history of each individual patient was recorded, followed by an oral and radiological examination.

Patients with a history of preprosthetic surgery (eg, augmentation procedures, vestibuloplasty), patients who previously had been treated with dental implants, and patients who were not suitable for dental implant treatment because of their medical condition, were excluded from this study. One third of patients received a mainly tissue-supported overdenture on two implants with ball attachments

(2IBA); one third received a combined implant-tissue–supported overdenture on two implants with a single bar (2ISB); and one third received a mainly implant-supported overdenture on four implants with a triple bar (4ITB). If a mandibular implant overdenture was the indicated treatment, patients were informed of the three possible implant-based treatment strategies. They also were informed of the treatment's expected benefits as well as the theoretical risks. The patients were asked if they would agree to undergo any of the three treatment modalities without prior knowledge of the chosen treatment, which would be revealed after the computed treatment allocation. The treatment allocation was calculated using a balancing procedure[15] aimed at ensuring an equal distribution of the patients over the treatment groups with regard to the administered balancing criteria: age, gender, the longevity of mandibular edentulousness, the number of previously worn mandibular dentures, the age of the present mandibular denture, the morphology of the maxilla and mandible, and the symphyseal bone height of the mandible measured on a lateral head plate.

These criteria were used in a computerized random allocation procedure with a group controller; the randomization procedure was carried out by a third party at an independent location. In this controlled manner, three statistically comparable randomized groups were created. The pretreatment comparability of the treatment groups was examined by an analysis of variance (one-way ANOVA). The surgeons and the prosthodontists were bound by the results, and the patients were treated accordingly.

Prosthetic Treatment

All implants were placed by an oral and maxillofacial surgeon using local anesthesia. No bone augmentation procedures or bone re-generation procedures were used. The sutures were removed 10 days postinsertion. During this period patients were not allowed to wear their mandibular dentures. Two weeks postinsertion, the existing mandibular denture was adapted to the mucosal tissues with a tissue conditioning material (Softliner, GC, Tokyo, Japan). In some cases this was repeated during the osseointegration phase due to wear of the tissue-conditioning material. Three months postinsertion, the maxillofacial prosthodontist began the manufacture of a new complete maxillary denture and a mandibular overdenture on either two or four implants; this phase was designated as *primary prosthetic treatment*. For an overdenture with ball attachments, a Dalla Bona matrix (Cendres et Métaux, Bienne, Switzerland) was used. The bars connecting the two or four implants in the other two groups were egg-shaped Dolder bars (Cendres et Métaux). In the case of two interconnected implants, one matrix (Cendres et Métaux) was used, and three corresponding matrices were used for a triple bar (Cendres et Métaux) and were incorporated into the overdenture. The dentures were manufactured for an optimal fit and balanced occlusion. None of the dentures were fitted with a precast metal reinforcement.

A minimum of six visits, including one recall visit, was required to complete treatment. For the treatment evaluation it was arbitrarily stated that primary prosthetic treatment ended 3 months after insertion of the new dentures. Visits to the clinic after this period (including the six monthly recalls) were defined as *aftercare*.

Oral Hygiene

Since the ITI dental implant system is a one-stage system, part of the implant is exposed to the oral flora at gingival level during osseointegration. Immediately after suture removal, patients received instructions on basic implant hygiene. Prior to that point, patients rinsed their mouths twice daily with a 0.2% chlorhexidine solution.

The patients visited the hygienist at least once during the osseointegration period to evaluate oral hygiene effectiveness. Peri-implant parameters were registered.[26] After the superstructure and new dentures had been placed by the prosthodontist, the patient was given additional instructions on controlling plaque around the superstructure and denture. The patient visited the hygienist every 12 to 26 weeks during the first year to ensure that oral hygiene was up to standard. The number of visits needed for the instruction and treatment was recorded.

Aftercare

Aftercare is defined as all care necessary during the periods from 3 to 16 months and from 16 to 96 months postinsertion of the dentures, including recalls every 6 months. Aftercare consisted of surgical, prosthetic, and/or oral hygiene measures taken to keep the peri-implant tissues healthy and to ensure optimal denture fit and occlusion. The time and costs involved in providing aftercare by the oral and maxillofacial surgeon, the prosthodontists, and the number of visits to the oral hygienist were recorded. Both time and costs, including those of the dental technician, were recorded. Care given up to 3 months postinsertion were recorded as part of the primary treatment.

Clinical Implant Performance Scale

In order to make a realistic comparison of different implant overdenture treatment modali-

ties, a clinical implant performance (CIP) scale was first used by Geertman et al in a clinical trial in which three implant systems supporting overdentures were compared.[17] The CIP scale considers all surgical, prosthetic, radiographic, and peri-implant problems and treatment needs that occurred from the day the dentures were inserted to, in this study, the evaluation period 19 months postinsertion. The CIP scale can be used when comparing perimucosal implant systems as well as transmandibular implant systems. Table 8-1 notes items and scores of the CIP scale for perimucosal implants recorded in the BIOS study.

The various factors considered important for clinical implant performance are scored on a five-point scale:

0 = Success, no complications
1 = Minor complications that do not need intervention or are easily treated
2 = Complications with a chance of recovery or stabilization of the present situation
3 = Serious complications that may lead to failure of the implant system
4 = Failure of the implant system

To calculate the x-ray score used in the CIP scale, radiographs taken at 19 months and at 8 years postinsertion were compared to those made immediately after primary treatment. The x-ray scores are classified as follows:

0 = No apparent bone loss around the implant
1 = Reduction of the bone level not exceeding one third of the implant length
2 = Reduction of the bone level between one third and one half of the implant length
3 = Reduction of the bone level exceeding one half of the implant length

Table 8-1 Items and scores in the CIP scale

Item No.	Problems and complications	CIP score 2IBA/2ISB	CIP score 4ITB
01	Broken abutment	1	1
02	Correction of hyperplastic mucosa around implant	1	1
03	Correction of nonfitting mesostructure	2	2
04	Broken mesostructure	2	2
05	Correction of occlusion and articulation	1	1
06	Loss of complete implant system	4	4
07	Loosening of one or more mesostructure screws	1	1
08	Reline maxillary or mandibular denture	1	1
09	Minor disturbance of mental nerve	1	1
10	Severe disturbance of mental nerve	2	2
11	Loosening of a clip or Dalla Bona matrix	1	1
12	Removal of one implant	4	3
13	Removal of two implants	4	3
14	Removal of three implants	4	4
15	x-ray score = 0, PD < 5.5 mm	0	0
16	x-ray score = 0, PD > 5.5 mm	1	1
17	x-ray score = 1, PD < 5.5 mm	1	1
18	x-ray score = 1, PD > 5.5 mm	2	2
19	x-ray score = 2, PD < 5.5 mm	2	2
20	x-ray score = 2, PD > 5.5 mm	3	3
21	x-ray score = 3, PD < 5.5 mm	3	3
22	x-ray score = 3, PD > 5.5 mm	3	3

(2IBA) Two-implant overdenture with ball attachment; (2ISB) two-implant bar-retained overdenture; (4ITB) four-implant overdenture with triple bar; (PD) probing depth.

Table 8-2 Patient responses (%) with respect to social functioning with complete dentures before (white rows) and 19 months after (shaded rows) treatment

With the denture I now wear, I feel comfortable . . .	Totally agree	Agree	No opinion	Disagree	Totally disagree
Visiting my family	13	57	10	16	4
	80	20	0	0	0
Visiting friends	18	50	8	19	5
	79	20	1	0	0
At parties	14	41	11	23	11
	77	20	1	2	0
Eating in a restaurant	11	31	4	35	19
	74	21	1	3	1

Patient Satisfaction

Many studies have shown that patients' opinions of implant-retained overdentures are more positive compared to their views of conventional dentures. At baseline, there were no differences among the three treatment groups in patients' complaints about their dentures. Nineteen months postinsertion of the implant-supported overdentures, there was a significant improvement in patient satisfaction and social functioning (Table 8-2). There also was significant pain reduction experienced by patients in the overdenture group. The same questions were asked again after 96 months. After 96 months, as after 19 months, there also was no statistical difference in comparison of the three treatment groups for the parameters mentioned above. There was, however, a significant slight decrease in the euphoric reactions when compared to those after 19 months. This decrease probably is caused by patients becoming more accustomed to their improved dental health. After 8 years, the 2ISB group showed the highest subjective retention rating.

Treatment Costs

Table 8-3 shows the total treatment costs during the first 19 months and also after 8 years postinsertion. The costs of the prosthetic treatment are calculated up to 19 months after denture placement and include dental laboratory costs. These results suggest that there is little difference between the 2IBA and 2ISB groups in this respect. The 4ITB treatment is nearly 40% more expensive than the least expensive treatment modality, 2IBA.

The time involved with prosthetic aftercare between 19 months and 96 months was not calculated in the total costs. Statistical analysis shows that there is no statistical difference be-

Table 8-3 Treatment costs during the 8-year evaluation period

	Total costs after 19 months (EUR)	Dental technician costs during 8 years (EUR)	Time involved with aftercare (min)	Total costs after 8 years (EUR)
2IBA	1,933	124	163	2,057
2ISB	2,084	120	175	2,204
4ITB	2,665	84	167	2,785

(2IBA) Two-implant overdenture with ball attachment; (2ISB) two-implant bar-retained overdenture; (4ITB) four-implant overdenture with triple bar.

Table 8-4 Distribution (%) of patients by number of aftercare visits per patient during 8 years (patients' initiative)

No. of visits	2IBA	2ISB	4ITB	Mean 2ISB/4ITB
0–4	30	60	72	66
5–8	40	18	18	18
> 9	30	21	9	15

(2IBA) Two-implant overdenture with ball attachment; (2ISB) two-implant bar-retained overdenture; (4ITB) four-implant overdenture with triple bar.

tween the 2IBA and 2ISB groups either in total costs or in time involved in prosthetic aftercare. The three groups show no difference in the time invested in the prosthetic aftercare (Kruskal-Wallis test).

Since there was no difference in the total time involved in the patient's aftercare when compared to the three treatment groups, the visits patients made to their clinic for aftercare during the 96-month follow-up period were evaluated. A differentiation was made between patient-initiated aftercare and aftercare concerning only reactivation of the retentive system. Table 8-4 demonstrates that the patients in the 2IBA group initiated more aftercare than

the 2ISB and 4ITB groups (2IBA versus 2ISB/4ITB; Kruskal-Wallis $P = .018$).

The number of visits per patient at which patients initiated reactivation of the retentive systems again demonstrates that patients in the 2IBA group required more aftercare than patients in the 2ISB and 4ITB groups (Table 8-5). The different treatment modalities were also compared with respect to the CIP scale. After the first 19-month evaluation period, the 4ITB group noted a CIP score greater than 2. This higher score involved six patients for whom the bone loss measured on radiographs indicated an x-ray score of 2 or greater[26] and a probing depth in excess of 5.5 mm. The 2ISB

Table 8-5 Distribution (%) of patients by number of visits per patient to reactivate the retentive system (patients' initiative)

No. of visits	2IBA*	2ISB	4ITB	Mean 2ISB/4ITB
0–2	73	94	97	95
3–4	17	6	3	5
> 5	10	0	0	0

(2IBA) Two-implant overdenture with ball attachment; (2ISB) two-implant bar-retained overdenture; (4ITB) four-implant overdenture with triple bar.
*The difference between 2IBA and 2ISB/4ITB is statistically significant; Kruskal-Wallis $P = .001$.

group had the lowest mean CIP score. The difference between the 2IBA and 2ISB groups is not statistically significant (chi-square test $P >$ .05); however, there is a significant difference between the 2IBA and 2ISB groups and the 4ITB group (chi-square test $P < .05$). After 8 years postinsertion, most patients moved from CIP scores of 0 to 1. The reason for this shift is cervical bone loss around the neck of the implant and necessary prosthetic aftercare. There still is no statistical difference in the CIP score among the three treatment groups.

An interesting phenomenon is the influence of smoking on CIP scores. Approximately 40% of the patient group were smokers. The patients who smoked had a significantly higher CIP score after 96 months than did the nonsmokers. The patients who smoked had a mean CIP score of 1.5 and the nonsmokers had a mean CIP score of 1.1; this is statistically significant (chi-square test $P = .027$). Of the eight patients in the study who had CIP scale scores of categories 3 ("serious complications that may lead to failure of the implant system") and 4 ("failure of the implant system"), six were smokers.

Cost Effectiveness

To evaluate the efficacy of the three different treatment modalities, the total clinical implant performance must be compared with the treatment costs. This comparison provides insight to the "value for money" of the different treatment modalities. The data for total costs in Euros for the first 8 years of treatment against the mean CIP score reveal that the 2ISB group costs are very similar to the 2IBA group costs, but scores significantly lower on the CIP scale. For this reason, after 96 months follow-up, the 2ISB treatment option is proven to be the most cost effective of the three evaluated treatment options.

Implications

The costs involved with dental treatment strategies vary per patient, hospital, and treatment provider. Other factors such as environmental costs, loss of the patient's productive working hours or spare time, the use of medication, and many more are even more difficult to calculate. Therefore in this study, these factors were included in the cost of treatment. The costs calculated in this study were the costs directly involved with the treatment and treatment providers. The calculations are valid for the treatment carried out in the Ignatius Teaching Hospital in Breda, The Netherlands, and can be used to compare the costs of the three different treatment strategies.

The costs involved with the prosthetic treatment (see Table 8-3) reveal a significant difference in the total costs (treatment costs plus costs charged by the dental laboratory). Two-implant overdentures with ball attachments appear to be the least expensive, which reflects the lower costs generated by the dental laboratory for this treatment strategy; there is no soldering and there are no additional costs for gold caps. On the other hand, the Dalla Bona anchors are more expensive than the clips for a Dolder bar. Treatment with four-implant overdentures with a triple bar is considerably more expensive than the two-implant, single-bar overdenture because of the additional two gold caps, Dolder bars, soldering, clips, and fee.

Two-implant overdentures with ball attachments required the most aftercare. Apparently more recall time has to be invested for patients to keep the overdenture up to hygienic standards and to keep the patients satisfied. Specifically, the retentive mechanism in the ball attachment group needed the most attention. During the 8-year evaluation period, the patients with Dalla Bona anchors (ball attachments) needed their dentures to be activated more frequently than the other two groups. This does not indicate that the total aftercare time was greater than for other groups, but that the patients made more (shorter) visits.

Summary

Treatment of the edentulous mandible with a four-implant–retained overdenture is significantly more expensive than treatment with two-implant overdentures. However, there are fewer costs involved with aftercare in the former treatment group during the 8-year follow-up. Further long-term evaluation is necessary to determine whether the four-implant–retained overdenture therapy continues to require less long-term aftercare.

During the 96-month period of this investigation, the two-implant bar-retained overdenture treatment appeared to be the most effective for edentulous patients when considering patient satisfaction, clinical implant performance, and cost effectiveness. Finally, patients who smoke are at a higher risk of complications when treated with mandibular implant overdentures.

References

1. Adell R, Lekholm U, Rockler B, Brånemark PI. A 15-year study of osseointegrated implants in the edentulous jaw. Int J Oral Surg 1981;10:387–416.
2. Adell R, Eriksson B, Lekholm U, Brånemark PI, Jemt T. A longterm follow-up study of osseointegrated implants in the treatment of the totally edentulous jaws. Int J Oral Maxillofac Implants 1990;5:347–359.
3. Adell R. Clinical results of osseointegrated implants supporting fixed prosthesis in edentulous jaws. J Prosthet Dent 1983;50:251–254.
4. Albrektsson T, Blomberg S, Brånemark A, Carlsson GE. Edentulousness—an oral handicap. Patient reactions to treatment with jawbone-anchored prostheses. J Oral Rehabil 1987;14:503–511.
5. Enquist B, Bergedal T, Kallus T, Linden U. A retrospective multicenter evaluation of osseointegrated implants supporting overdentures. Int J Oral Maxillofac Implants 1988;3:129–134.

6. Adell R, Eriksson B, Lekholm U, Brånemark PI, Jemt T. A long-term follow-up study of osseointegrated implants in the treatment of totally edentulous jaws. Int J Oral Maxillofac Implants 1990;5:347–359.

7. Bosker H, van Dijk L. The transmandibular implant: a 12-year follow-up study. J Oral Maxillofac Surg 1989; 47:442–450.

8. Zarb GA, Schmitt A. The longitudinal clinical effectiveness of osseointegrated dental implants: The Toronto study. Part I: Surgical results. J Prosthet Dent 1990;63:451–457.

9. Naert I, De Clercq M, Theuniers G, Schepers E. Overdentures supported by osseointegrated fixtures for the edentulous mandible: A 2.5-year report. Int J Oral Maxillofac Implants 1988;3:191–196.

10. Mericske-Stern R. Clinical evaluation of overdenture restorations supported by osseointegrated titanium implants: A retrospective study. Int J Oral Maxillofac Implants 1990;5:375–383.

11. Johns RB, Jemt T, Heath MR, Hutton JE, et al. A multicenter study of overdentures supported by Brånemark implants. Int J Oral Maxillofac Implants 1992; 7:162–167.

12. Wismeijer D, Vermeeren JIJF, van Waas MAJ. Patient satisfaction with overdentures supported by one-stage TPS implants. Int J Oral Maxillofac Implants 1992;7:51–55.

13. Wismeijer D, Vermeeren JIJF, van Waas MAJ. A 6.5-year evaluation of patient satisfaction and prosthetic aftercare in patient treatment using overdentures supported by ITI-implants. Int J Oral Maxillofac Implants 1995;10:744–749.

14. Cune MS. Overdentures on Dental Implants. [thesis]. Utrecht, the Netherlands: University of Utrecht, 1993.

15. Kapur KK, Garrett NR. Requirements for clinical trials. J Dent Educ 1988;52:760–764.

16. Esposito M, et al. Quality assessment of randomized controlled trials of oral implants. Int J Oral Maxillofac Implants 2001;16:783–792.

17. Geertman ME, Boerrigter EM, van't Hof MA, et al. Clinical aspects of a multicenter clinical trial of implant-retained mandibular overdentures in patients with severely resorbed mandibles. J Prost Dent 1996;75:194-204.

18. Feine JS, de Grandmont P, Boudrias P, et al. Within-subject comparisons of implant-supported mandibular prothesis: Choice of prosthesis. J Dent Res 1994;73:1105–1111.

19. Burns DR, Unger JW, Elswick RK Jr, Giglio JA. Prospective clinical evaluation of mandibular implant overdentures: Part I: Retention, stability and tissue response. J Prost Dent 1995;73:354–363.

20. Davis DM, Rogers JO, Packer ME. The extent of maintenance required by implant-retained mandibular overdentures: A 3-year report. Int J Oral Maxillofac Implants 1996;11:767–774.

21. Batenburg RHK, van Oort RP, Reintsema H, Brouwer TT, Raghoebar GM, Boering G. Mandibular overdentures supported by two Branemark, IMZ, or ITI implants. A prospective comparative preliminary study: One-year results. Clin Oral Implants Res 1998;9:374–383.

22. Bergendal T, Engquist B. Implant-supported overdentures: A longitudinal prospective study. Int J Oral Maxillofac Implants 1998;13:253–262.

23. Fontijn-Teekamp FA, Slagter AP, van't Hof MA, Geertman MA, Kalk WA. Bite forces with mandibular implant-retained overdentures. J Dent Res 1998; 77:1832–1839.

24. Garrett NR, Kapur KK, Hamada MO, et al. A randomized clinical trial comparing the efficacy of mandibular implant-supported overdentures and conventional dentures in diabetic patients. Part II. Comparisons of masticatory performance. J Prosthet Dent 1998;79:632–640.

25. Wismeijer D, Van Waas MAJ, Vermeeren JIJF, Mulder J, Kalk W. Patient satisfaction with implant-supported mandibular overdentures. A comparison of three treatment strategies on ITI-dental implants. Int J Oral Maxillofac Surg 1997;26:263–267.

26. Wismeijer D, Van Waas MAJ, Vermeeren JIJF, Mulder J, Kalk W. Clinical and radiological results of patients treated with three treatment modalities for overdentures on implants of the ITI-dental implant system. Clin Oral Implants Res 1999:10:297–306.

CHAPTER 9

Indications and Treatment Planning for Mandibular Implant Overdentures

Thomas D. Taylor

Planning a patient's mandibular overdenture treatment is a straightforward process that will yield very predictable results if done in a systematic manner. This treatment planning process is reviewed in detail in this chapter.

It is no longer a safe assumption that patients who are treated with implant-supported overdentures were first introduced to the concept by their dentist. As dental implant therapy becomes more common, denture wearers are increasingly aware that there is an alternative to the mucosa-supported complete mandibular denture and frequently seek information about implant alternatives. It is becoming more important for clinicians who offer complete denture services to also offer dental implants as a means of increasing patient satisfaction and improving quality of life. The process of evaluating an edentulous patient for dental implant therapy is straightforward and extremely satisfying to both patient and provider.

Initial Consultation

At the initial consultation, the clinician can determine whether the patient already has well-constructed, functional dentures that would serve adequately by the addition of two implants in the anterior mandible to stabilize and retain the denture. Generally it is not advisable for a clinician to undertake the modification of a mandibular complete denture into an overdenture unless the same clinician originally provided the dentures. It is best to avoid working with dentures made by another clinician, particularly when entering into an implant treatment plan.

Initial discussions with a patient regarding a proposed treatment plan that involves the placement of dental implants for overdenture support must take into consideration the patient's current dental status and concerns. Many times, the patient who has had experience with complete dentures is enthusiastic about any procedure that may improve the comfort and function of a mandibular denture. In other situations, the patient may be satisfied, or nearly so, with a mandibular complete denture, and the possibility of improved comfort and function is not a high priority. The dentist must be aware of patient concerns and approach the treatment planning discussion from a conservative direction. Treatment with an implant-supported denture should not be pursued for patients who are not confident that the process is appropriate for their needs.

For the patient facing edentulism in the mandible for the first time, the decision to proceed immediately to an implant overdenture may be difficult. Frequently, the patient already has had experience with a maxillary complete denture, and the quality of that experience will influence the patient's decision whether to proceed with conventional complete denture fabrication for the mandibular arch or to place implants at the time of extraction. The latter option minimizes the healing period before an overdenture or a fixed implant-supported prosthesis can be placed. A patient who has been satisfied with a maxillary complete denture may prefer to try the conventional mandibular denture before committing to the additional expense and surgery involved with implant placement. Unlike implant placement in a partially edentulous patient, particularly in esthetic areas of the mouth, delayed implant placement in an edentulous mandible does not compromise the predictability or quality of the result. It can be argued that a moderately resorbed mandible is preferable for implant placement when compared to the newly edentate mandible with a prominent alveolar ridge in the anterior region. Implant placement and fabrication of an overdenture attachment system, either bar or ball type, is much more difficult in the minimally resorbed mandible because of a lack of available space within the profile of the denture. In such instances, the likelihood of denture fracture due to insufficient bulk of denture base material may be problematic.

Another potential argument for deferred implant placement is that it gives the patient the experience of wearing a complete denture without overdenture anchorage. This makes the experience of gaining additional support, retention, and stability with overdenture anchorage a more dramatic and satisfying change. The decision to use immediate or delayed implant placement for overdenture anchorage should be made on a patient-by-patient basis.

The determination of whether a mandibular implant-assisted overdenture is appropriate for a patient must be made regardless of whether a preexisting denture will be modified to receive implants or whether the patient requires fabrication of new maxillary and mandibular denture prostheses in conjunction with dental implant therapy.

Successful implant overdenture therapy is dependent on adherence to basic principles of denture fabrication, as is treatment with conventional complete dentures. Adequate denture base extension and adaptation to the underlying soft tissues are prerequisites for success. The assumption that the additional stability and retention provided by the implants will compensate for less-than-adequate denture base support will likely limit the successful outcome of treatment and may lead to problems with patient acceptance and comfort, as well as chronic denture base irritation and accelerated alveolar resorption. It is important to take time to determine the proper vertical dimension of occlusion, accurate registration of centric relation, and proper tooth position within the arches. Less-than-ideal registration of any of these factors may lead to ongoing denture instability, soreness, and patient dissatisfaction. In short, the use of dental implants to overcome or mask deficiencies in denture fabrication may result in an unsatisfactory outcome and treatment failure.

Consideration of Overall Patient Health for Implant Surgery

There are surprisingly few absolute contraindications for dental implant placement. As a general rule, any medical condition that contraindicates elective surgery of any kind may be considered a contraindication for dental implant surgery. Placement of dental implants, particularly in the edentulous anterior mandible, is a straightforward procedure with few anatomic risks and a low morbidity rate.

Many candidates for dental implant surgery are elderly, and their overall medical condition may be complex. Consultation with the patient's physician is important to ensure that surgical risks are minimized. It cannot be assumed that the physician will be aware of exactly what is involved with surgical placement of dental implants, and physician education may become part of the treatment planning process. The surgical risk of implant surgery in the medically compromised patient may be offset by the potential increase in function, food selection, and quality of life that could result from treatment with an implant overdenture. Adjustment of daily medications that affect hemostasis may by suggested for patients on long-term anticoagulant therapy, which can include the low-dosage aspirin regimen that is routinely prescribed for many older patients.

Medical conditions that are generally considered contraindications for dental implant placement include uncontrolled diabetes or other metabolic diseases that alter the normal healing process, previous radiation therapy to the oral cavity (although with careful management this is not an absolute contraindication), hematologic and immunologic diseases that put the patient at risk for minor surgical procedures, and chronic use of systemic steroids.

Systemic steroid use in particular is a substantial risk factor for successful osseointegration of dental implants. Neither age nor osteoporosis have been shown to be contraindications for successful dental implant osseointegration.[1] Care should be taken with patients who have severe osteoporosis, due to the increased risk of fracture resulting from the surgical osteotomy and loading of a potentially weakened mandible.

An additional relative contraindication is tobacco use. While the literature is not conclusive as to the effect of smoking on the success of dental implant treatment, there is strong evidence that heavy tobacco use severely compromises dental implant therapy.[2] Tobacco use has been implicated in both early (failure to integrate) and delayed (peri-implant infection) implant loss. The question that must be addressed with a patient who smokes is whether that patient is willing to accept complete responsibility for the increased risk of failure to the extent of being willing to pay for and undergo the procedure with no guarantees of success. If the patient understands and accepts the potential increased risk, then implant therapy can proceed as planned. Obviously, a smoking cessation program prior to surgery would likely increase the chances of successful treatment.

Radiographic Examination of the Edentulous Mandible

The panoramic radiograph is the most convenient and readily available radiographic examination tool when considering dental implant placement. Frequently, the clinician who initially evaluates an edentulous patient for possible treatment with an implant-assisted overdenture is a general dentist or prosthodontist. In this situation, a panoramic radiograph will assist

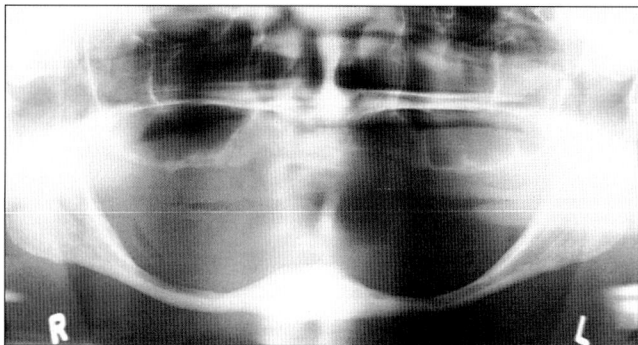

Fig 9-1 The panoramic radiograph is a useful screening film for evaluation of the edentulous mandible when planning for implant overdentures. Caution should be exercised, however, when evaluating structures near the midline, as distortion and magnification tend to be maximized in this area.

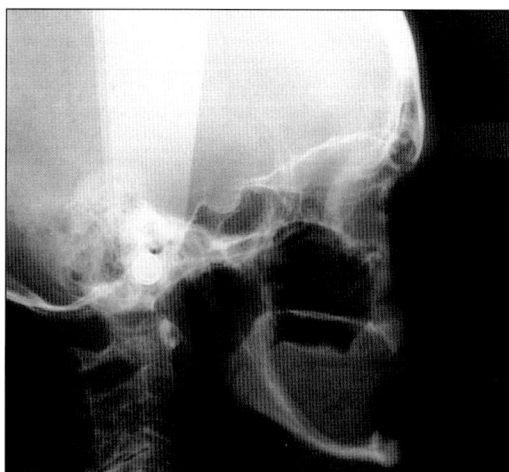

Fig 9-2 The lateral cephalometric radiograph is ideal for evaluating the residual mandible in preparation for implant placement in the anterior region. Distortion and magnification are minimized and the symphyseal region is represented in an anatomically accurate form. This is the same patient seen in Fig 9-1. Distortion of the panoramic film is obvious.

planning and is useful to evaluate residual pathologic lesions of the jaws and to judge the amount of residual bone available for implant placement (Fig 9-1). While a panoramic radiograph is subject to substantial distortion of the image, it still is an acceptable film to initially gauge the amount of residual bone. Additional radiographic analysis, when necessary, should be performed at the discretion of the surgeon placing the implants. The lateral cephalometric view gives an excellent cross-sectional view of the anterior mandible in the symphyseal region (Fig 9-2). This view provides information about the labiolingual thickness of the mandible, the presence of concavities in the lower part of

the mandible, and the quality of bone present. The lateral cephalometric radiograph is more accurate than the panoramic radiograph for imaging the symphyseal region. It is relatively inexpensive and requires minimal radiation exposure. Similarly, an occlusal radiograph may be useful to determine labiolingual mandibular thickness (Fig 9-3). Tomographic and computerized tomographic (CT) surveys, while frequently necessary in other areas of the jaws for implant planning, are rarely necessary in the edentulous anterior mandible. It bears repeating that radiographic examination beyond an initial panoramic view is at the discretion of the surgeon placing the implants.

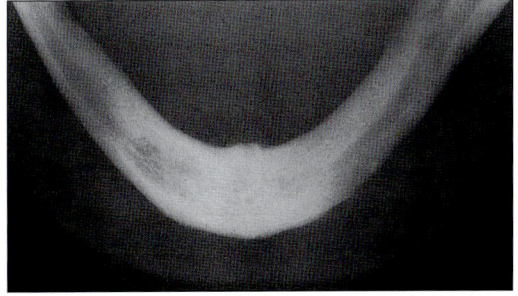

Fig 9-3 An occlusal radiograph is useful to evaluate the labiolingual thickness of the mandible in the interforaminal region. When done properly, this view provides accurate information with minimal distortion or magnification. This is the same patient seen in Figs 9-1 and 9-2.

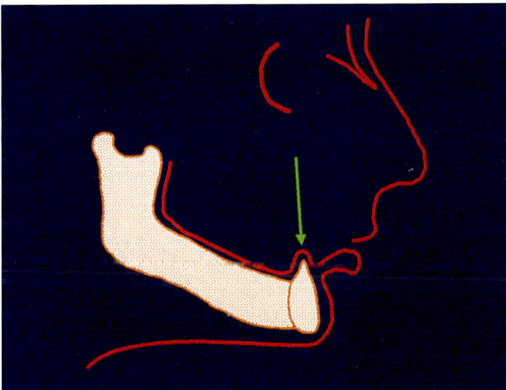

Fig 9-4a A knife-edge ridge seen clinically may cause concern regarding the availability of adequate bone thickness for implant placement. The occlusal and lateral cephalometric films will assist in determining the actual width of bone available.

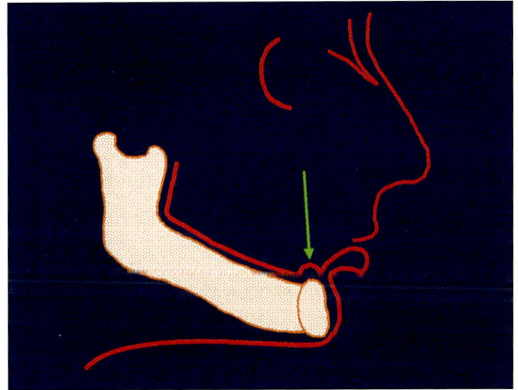

Fig 9-4b Minimal to moderate alveolectomy at the time of implant placement eliminates that portion of the alveolar ridge that is of inadequate labiolingual width for implant placement. In situations where there has been minimal postextraction resorption in the anterior mandible, moderate alveolectomy also permits implant placement in a more apical position, thereby increasing the space available for the overdenture attachment components. Space is gained at the expense of the alveolar process.

Clinical examination initially may lead to the determination that the labiolingual thickness of the mandible is inadequate to permit implant placement. In this situation, the lateral cephalometric and/or occlusal views are useful to gauge the actual thickness of the intersymphyseal mandible. Judicious crestal alveolectomy at the time of surgery frequently can eliminate the narrow, knife-edge portion of the residual alveolus and may allow implant placement into the broader basal bone (Figs 9-4a and 9-4b). It is rare to find a mandible with a basal area of insufficient labiolingual thickness for placement of standard-diameter implants. The need for

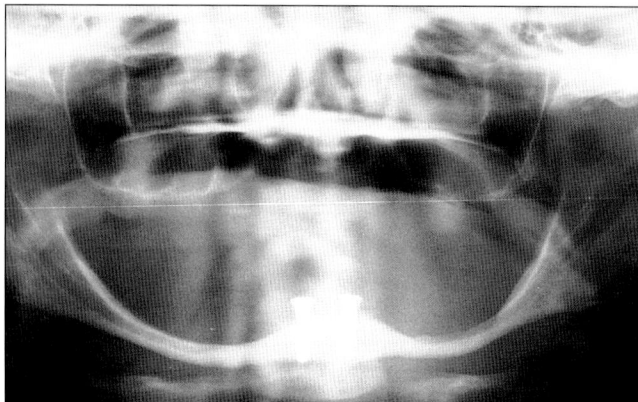

Fig 9-5a Two implants have been placed into this severely resorbed mandible (same patient seen in Figs 9-1 to 9-3). The tips of the implants penetrate the inferior border of the anterior mandible. This allows for the superior portion of the implants to be placed in an ideal position relative to the residual mandible. Deposition of bone around the apices of implants placed in this manner is seen frequently in radiographs taken after the implants have been in function for a period of time.

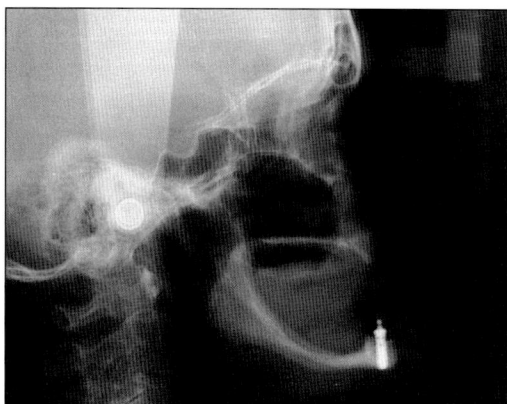

Fig 9-5b The implants with ball anchor abutments attached are in an ideal position for overdenture fabrication (same patient as in Fig 9-5a).

alveolectomy and the associated reduction in mandibular height should be evaluated and planned for by the surgeon and the clinician fabricating the denture prior to surgery. Modest reduction of the height of the anterior alveolar process also may be beneficial in creating additional vertical thickness or space for the final denture. This facilitates placement of the retentive bar and attachments within the confines of the denture base without necessitating overbulking of the denture.

The minimal amount of vertical mandibular height necessary for implant placement in the anterior edentulous mandible is the subject of some debate. Some clinicians advocate surgical augmentation of the mandible in preparation for implant placement. Other clinicians feel that as little as 5 to 7 mm of vertical bone height is sufficient for implant placement. Penetration of the inferior cortex and placement of the implant with its tip extending beyond the inferior border of the mandible has been successfully

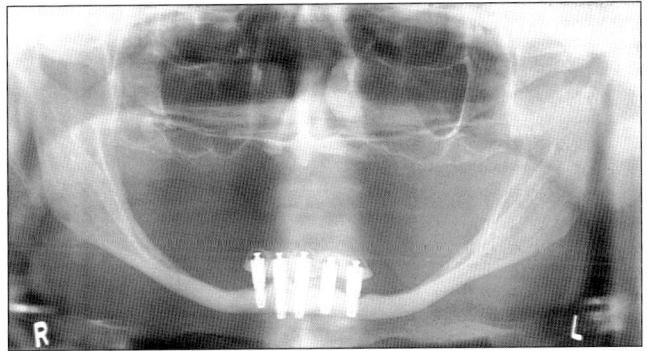

Fig 9-6a A severely resorbed mandible in a patient who is being considered for implant placement.

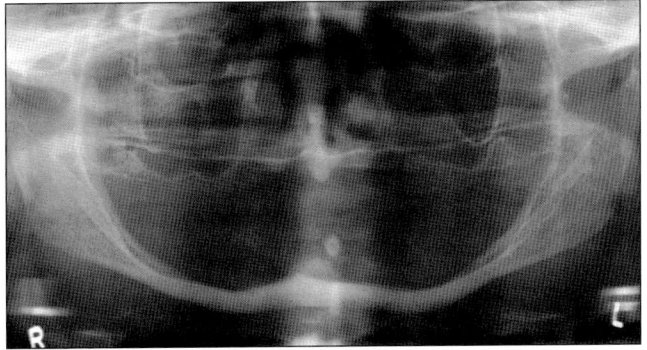

Fig 9-6b Five interforaminal implants have been placed in the anterior mandible of the patient seen in Fig 9-6a. Extension of the implant tips beyond the inferior border allowed this patient to be treated without mandibular augmentation through bone grafting.

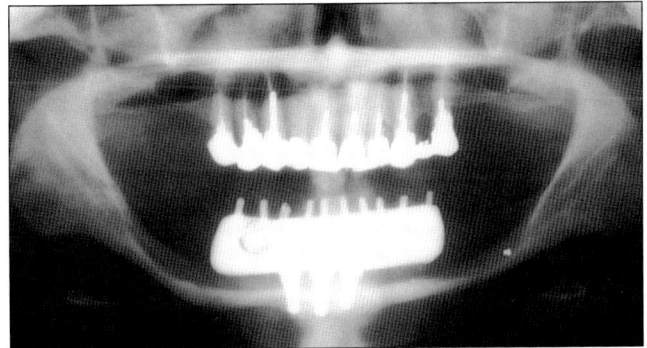

Fig 9-7 A mandibular fixed-detachable cantilever prosthesis placed on three 6-mm single-stage implants. The prosthesis functioned successfully against opposing natural teeth. There is evidence of alveolar ridge growth in the posterior mandible at 3 years postinsertion. (Courtesy of Dr Mats Hallman, Gavle, Sweden.)

performed for many years. The added cost, increased treatment time, complexity, and potential morbidity of vertical ridge augmentation should be carefully considered before proceeding. There currently is no evidence that longer implants placed into augmented ridges are more likely to succeed than short implants placed in minimal residual bone (Figs 9-5 to 9-7).

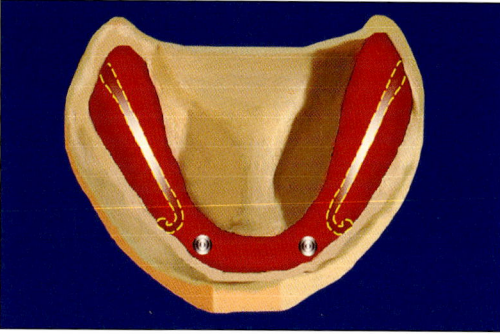

Fig 9-8 Traditional placement of dental implants for a mandibular overdenture. The placement of the implants in the canine positions may preclude future placement of implants between these and the mental foramina should the patient desire additional implant treatment.

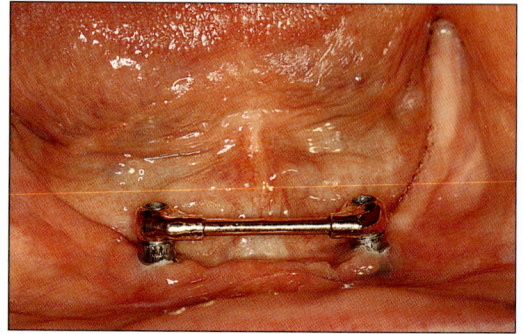

Fig 9-9 A splinted bar between two implants in the canine positions must be cantilevered to the anterior to avoid impingement on the tongue space by the overdenture. This anterior cantilever may create bending moments for the implant pillars, which could cause component failure through loosening or fracture following functional loading.

Site Selection for Implant Placement

Determination of implant number and position should be the decision of the clinician fabricating the overdenture, rather than that of the surgeon placing the implants. Four implants placed anterior to the mental foramina are frequently used for overdenture fabrication. An overdenture placed over four widely spaced implants is likely to be fully implant-supported during functional loading. The ability to gain soft tissue support in addition to implant support is difficult, and with even the slightest settling of the prosthesis following placement, the implants assume the support of the entire denture. Four implants are sufficient in most cases to support a fixed-detachable type of prosthesis, which precludes the need for overdenture support and reduces maintenance problems associated with nonparallel bar-and-clip overdenture designs.

The most straightforward use of dental implants as overdenture abutments is with two implants placed symmetrically in the anterior mandible. Frequently these are placed in the position of the canine teeth (Fig 9-8). Selection of the canine position for implant placement perhaps is the result of clinicians' experience with overdentures supported by natural teeth. The mandibular canines frequently are the last natural teeth remaining and are useful as overdenture abutments. However, it is important to consider whether the canine position is best suited for implant placement. The argument for moving slightly anterior, to the lateral incisor position, has several advantages. Placement of two implants in the canine positions frequently requires that a connecting bar, when used, be cantilevered to the anterior to avoid encroaching on the tongue space and floor of the mouth. This is particularly important in a situation with a tapering arch form. This complicates the design of the bar and may increase the risk

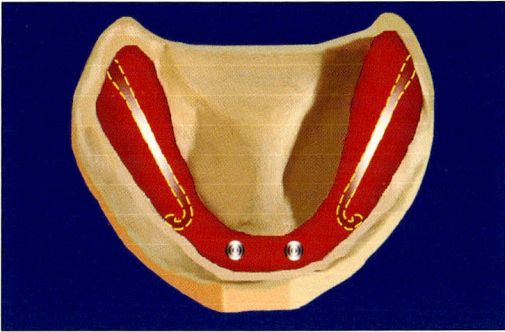

Fig 9-10a Placement of two implants in the lateral incisor positions (about 14 to 15 mm center to center) allows for future placement of implants to the posterior should the patient desire additional implant therapy.

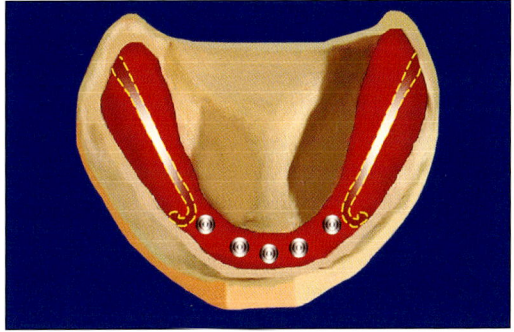

Fig 9-10b Placement of three additional implants is feasible when the original two implants are placed in the lateral incisor positions.

of screw loosening or fracture due to bending moments involved with cantilever loading (Fig 9-9). Implant placement slightly more to the anterior reduces the potential need for off-center bar placement.

Placement of two implants in the lateral incisor position (approximately 14 to 15 mm center to center) does not preclude the possibility of placing additional implants more to the posterior if the patient subsequently wishes to be treated with a fixed-detachable, cantilever (hybrid) prosthesis (Figs 9-10a and 9-10b). If implants are placed in the canine position in a severely resorbed mandible, there may not be sufficient space anterior to the mental foramina for subsequent placement of additional implants with an adequate anterior-posterior spread to support a fixed-detachable prosthesis (see Fig 9-9). Placement of two implants in the lateral incisor positions allows sufficient space posterior to the implants and anterior to the mental foramina for additional implants. There also is adequate space for a fifth midline implant.

Another advantage of a more anterior placement of the two implant overdenture abutments is that this placement reduces the tendency for the mandibular denture to rotate around the fulcrum created between the two implant abutments. If the implants are placed in the canine position, there may be a tendency for the distal denture bases to lift when the patient incises with the anterior teeth. This is particularly problematic when the retentive components of the overdenture attachment system are designed to permit rotational freedom of movement around the implant fulcrum. Implant placement in the lateral incisor position reduces the anteroposterior distance from the incisal edges to the rotational axis between the implants, which reduces the tendency for the denture to lift to the posterior and thereby increases its stability (Figs 9-11a and 9-11b).

An additional important factor is the space needed for the retentive components. Sufficient interimplant space must be maintained, particularly when a bar-and-clip type of attach-

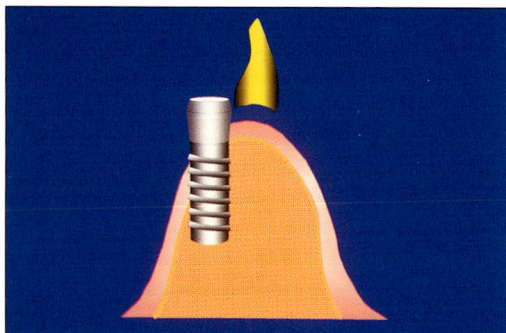

Fig 9-11a Placement of two implants in the canine positions places the potential fulcrum between the implants at some distance posterior to the incisal position of the anterior teeth. This may be particularly problematic for the patient with a tapered arch form, where the canine position is farther posterior than would be seen in a square arch form. It may also result in rotational instability of the overdenture when the patient attempts to incise food.

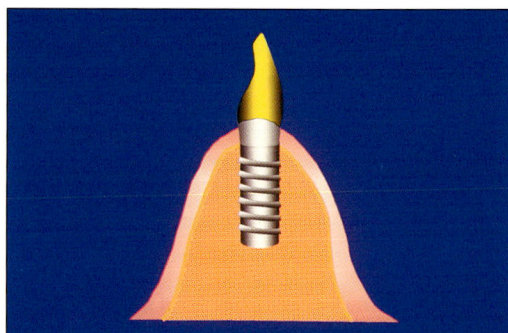

Fig 9-11b Positioning the implants and the resultant fulcrum more to the anterior (lateral incisor position) reduces the tendency for the posterior extensions of the overdenture to lift during incising.

ment is planned. An advantage of the non-splinted ball-anchor connection is that it is not as critical to maintain a large space between implants.

The use of a single midline implant as an overdenture abutment to increase mandibular denture retention and stability is a treatment modality worth further study. A single implant may be nearly as effective as two anterior implants in this regard and could reduce treatment cost considerably.[3,4]

Fabrication and Use of a Surgical Guide

While use of a surgical guide for placement of implants to support mandibular overdentures may seem unnecessary to some, it is beneficial in ensuring the predictable placement of the implants in the most usable position. A surgical guide should communicate the restorative dentist's choice for implant position to the sur-

geon with sufficient detail to prevent inadvertent malpositioning of the implants. The surgical guide is critical to successful completion of the proposed treatment plan and avoids miscommunication of the preferred position of the implants.

A surgical guide for the edentulous mandible is most frequently fabricated by duplicating the patient's existing mandibular complete denture. If an acceptable denture is not available, a trial denture that includes the correct vertical and horizontal jaw relationships and tooth position must be fabricated and duplicated for the surgical guide. The surgical guide must reflect the restorative dentist's preferred implant positions. A surgical guide that has the entire lingual portion of the denture open effectively provides information only about the labial contours of the denture (Fig 9-12). A more limiting design that specifically locates the desired implant positions should be provided to the surgeon (Fig 9-13).

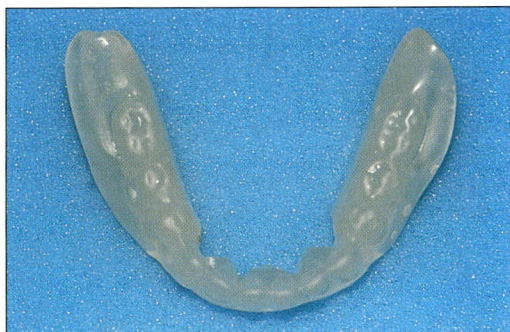

Fig 9-12 Surgical guide fabricated from a duplicated mandibular denture. While this design limits the surgical placement of implants in the labial direction, it does not preclude placing the implant too far to the lingual. It also does not insure that the implant will placed in the most desirable position around the arch.

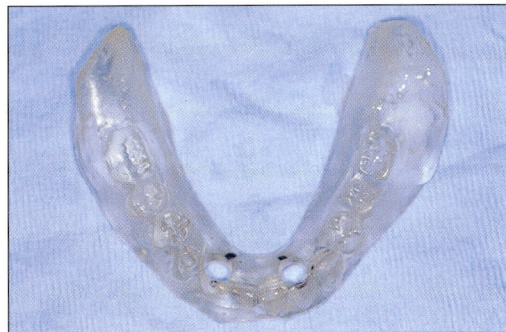

Fig 9-13 A surgical guide with large (5 to 6 mm) holes for drill access. This design limits placement in all directions and, if used, prevents less than optimal implant positioning.

Summary

Diagnostic and treatment planning steps for treatment with implant overdentures have been reviewed. Following an initial consultation to determine the patient's treatment needs and health status, the clinician should determine the amount of residual bone available for implant placement. Panoramic radiographs are ideal for this diagnosis. Lateral radiographs can be used at the discretion of the surgeon. Implant position requires careful planning prior to surgery. While two implants in the canine positions are common, placement in the lateral incisor positions provides increased denture stability and allows for future placement of additional implants if desired. Use of a surgical guide will ensure accurate placement.

The two-implant overdenture is a valuable therapeutic device that can be offered to all but the most severely physically debilitated edentulous patients. Implant overdentures clearly improve function, comfort, and quality of life for edentulous patients. Efforts to make this service financially attainable to more patients should be a top priority of the dental profession in the twenty-first century.

References

1. Meijer HJA, Batenburg HK, Raghoebar GM. Influence of patient age on the success rate of dental implants supporting an overdenture in an edentulous mandible: A 3-year prospective study. Int J Oral Maxillofac Implants 2001;16:522–526.
2. Quirynen M, Peeters W, Naert I, Coucke W, van Steenberghe D. Peri-implant health around screw-shaped CP titanium machined implants in partially edentulous patients with or without ongoing periodontitis. Clin Oral Implants Res 2001;12:589–594.
3. Krennmair G, Ulm C. The symphyseal single tooth implant for anchorage of a mandibular complete denture in geriatric patients: A clinical report. Int J Oral Maxillofac Implants 2001;16:98–104.
4. Cordioli G, Majzoub Z, Castagna S. Mandibular overdentures anchored to single implants: A five-year prospective study. J Prosthet Dent 1997;78:159–165.

CHAPTER 10

Prosthodontic Management of Maxillary and Mandibular Overdentures

Regina Mericske-Stern

Implants have had a significant impact on current prosthodontic treatment of edentulous patients. As a result of the development of osseointegrated dental implants, new treatment options have become available and new prosthetic designs have emerged. The use of implants under standard conditions has resulted in low morbidity in various indications. Valid clinical strategies for implant technology exist to ensure the quality of prosthetic reconstruction.

Osseointegrated techniques originally were intended to restore the edentulous arch with fixed prostheses; however, the current need for overdentures is reflected in numerous studies.

To this end, the main objective of implants placed in the edentulous arch is either (1) to avoid removable complete dentures by placement of implant-supported fixed prostheses or (2) to stabilize complete dentures by placement of implant-retained overdentures.

Local anatomic and morphologic conditions and general patient-related factors determine the choice of prosthesis. Generally, more implants are required for support of fixed prostheses than for overdentures. Therefore, the indication for fixed prostheses may be limited due to inadequate quantity and structure of the bone. Managing advanced ridge resorption often requires additional surgical procedures such as bone augmentation or other techniques to enhance local bone quantity. This is particularly true for the maxilla; such invasive methods require more specific patient selection than is needed for simple implant-prosthodontic procedures of the edentulous mandible. Even in the case of advanced atrophy, a standard surgical and prosthodontic protocol for placement of multiple (usually two) intraforaminal implants for overdenture support can mostly be used.

While several treatment alternatives with or without implants are available for the partially edentulous patient, until recently, conventional complete dentures were the only treatment option that could be offered to the completely edentulous patient. Thus, these patients were targeted to receive implants. Edentulous arches are prevalent mostly in older adults. There is solid evidence that implants placed in elderly patients have a similar prognosis as those placed in younger patients; however, advanced age is still considered by some to be a contraindication for implant placement.

A wide variety of implant systems have been developed and evaluated in clinical trials and reports, but a scientific background and well-

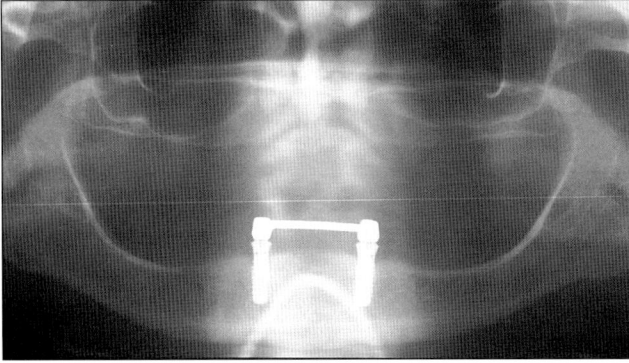

Fig 10-1a Two implants connected by a bar in a patient with osteoporosis with loose bone structure.

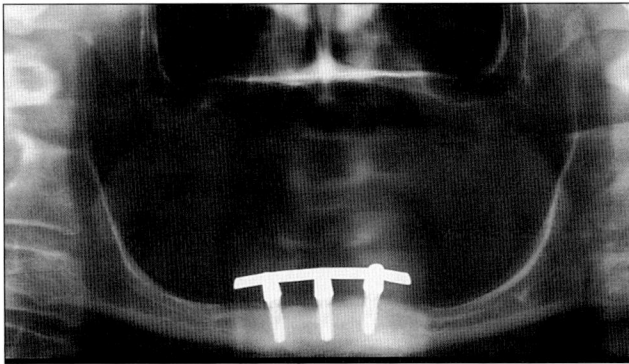

Fig 10-1b Three implants connected by a bar in a patient with advanced atrophy. The implants are 6-mm long.

designed studies are still often missing. Only a few implant systems and related prosthodontic treatments have been the subject of systematic investigations with proper study designs and can demonstrate scientifically and clinically reliable results. The aim of this chapter is to summarize developments of the overdenture treatment modality as compared to fixed prostheses, to discuss clinical and technical concepts, and to evaluate treatment outcomes.

Fixed Prostheses Versus Overdentures

Treatment with implants was originally aimed at providing the edentulous patient with fixed prostheses in the mandible and maxilla.[1] In the 1980s, the use of four implants with a connecting bar supporting an overdenture became a favored treatment modality and was recommended for the edentulous mandible. However, treatment protocols were not well established and its clinical efficacy was not yet documented by well-designed studies. The workshop on overdentures conducted by the University of Leuven in 1988 demonstrated the increasing interest in mandibular overdentures as opposed to fixed prostheses. At that time, studies suggesting the use of only two intraforaminal implants[2] to support mandibular overdentures were rare. Eventually this treatment concept gained acceptance, and today there is a clear trend to place only a few implants to support a mandibular prosthesis (Figs 10-1a and 10-1b).

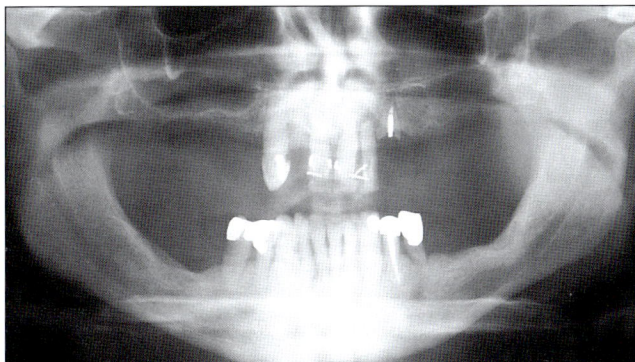

Fig 10-2a Residual dentition in the maxilla that cannot be maintained.

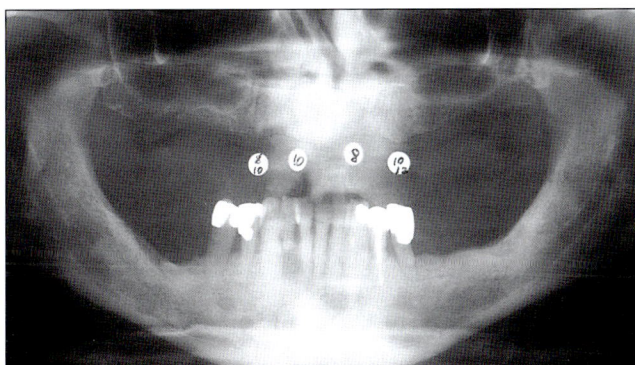

Fig 10-2b Note the large extension of the sinus.

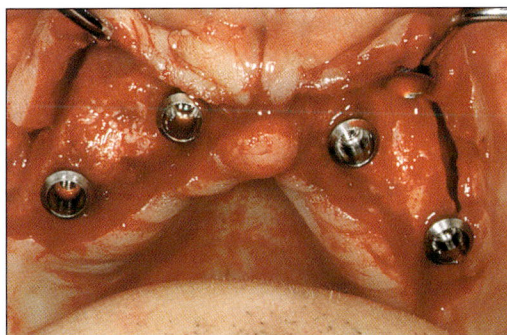

Fig 10-2c Four implants are well distributed in the anterior segment for overdenture support.

Results from a multicenter study in the late 1990s[3] showed that mandibular overdentures were the most frequently used treatment modality, constituting close to 50% of all implant therapy provided, while only 3% of all implants placed were used for maxillary overdentures. Nonetheless, advantages of maxillary overdentures are many compared to fixed prostheses. Implants often can be placed in the anterior segment of the maxillary jaw between the first premolars, avoiding interference with the sinuses (Figs 10-2a to 10-2c). Congruence of the position of implants and prosthetic teeth is not necessary, facilitating management of es-

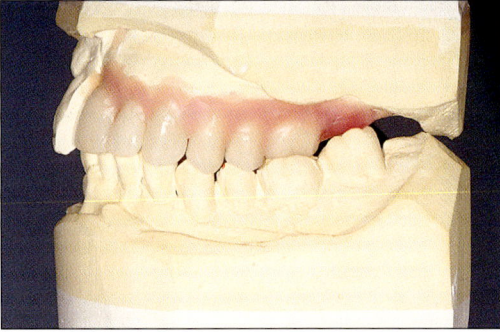
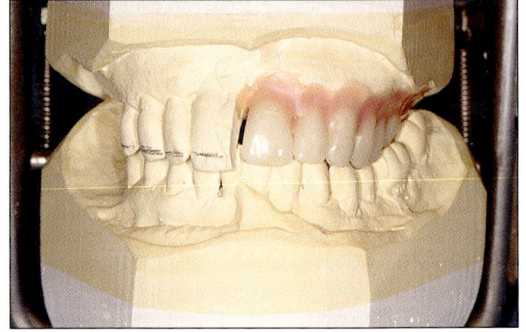

Figs 10-3a and 10-3b Tooth setup in the articulator shows desired esthetic corrections.

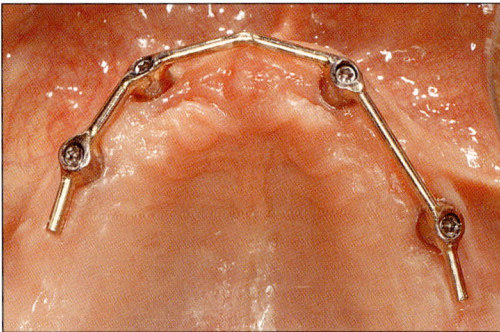
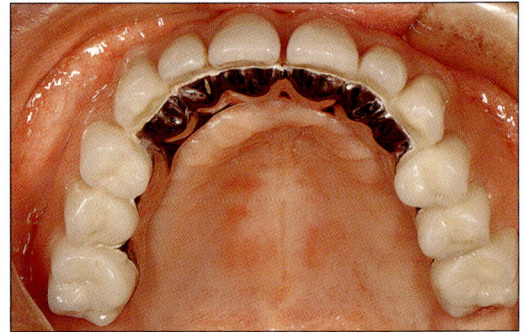

Figs 10-3c and 10-3d Congruent position of the implants and prosthetic teeth is not necessary.

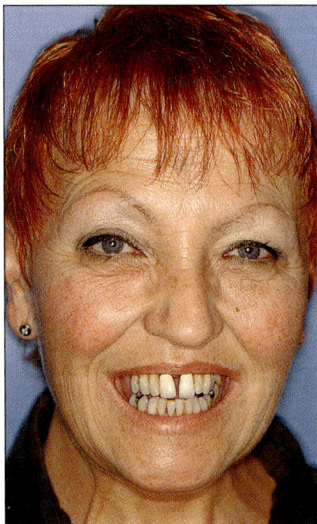
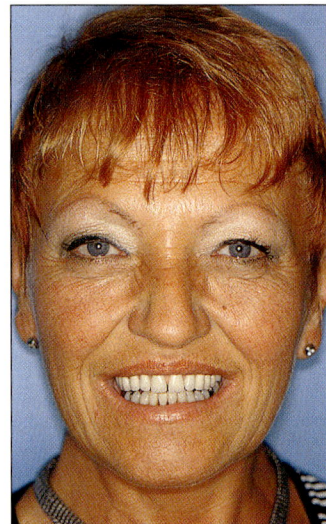

Figs 10-3e and 10-3f The patient before treatment *(left)* and after treatment with implant-supported overdentures *(right)*. Her appearance and esthetics have significantly improved.

thetic concerns, such as tooth position, soft tissue contour, facial morphology, and facial support (Figs 10-3a to 10-3f). Comparisons between fixed and removable prostheses in the maxilla suggest the use of four implants for overdenture support and a minimum of six implants for fixed prostheses.[4]

Sequelae of Tooth Loss and Wear of Complete Dentures

Sequelae of multiple tooth loss and edentulous arches include residual ridge resorption, orofacial collapse, impaired oral function, vulnerable tissues, and psychosocial impact. Pronounced loss of the residual ridge seen in the first year after tooth extraction becomes more moderate during the following years, but may vary from patient to patient. In many edentulous patients, esthetic appearance and function may be restored sufficiently with complete dentures, but stability and retention of complete dentures can be poor, particularly in the mandible. Tooth loss may have a noticeable psychosocial impact on the patient as well. Thus, the fixation of prostheses with implants has a great impact on prosthetic privacy, function, confidence in social activities (such as eating, speaking, laughing, and sports), and overall self-esteem.

A study[5] of edentulous patients' satisfaction and complaints about the impaired function of their mandibular complete dentures established a correlation between denture satisfaction and degree of atrophy. The number of complaints increased significantly with patients who had lost more than 50% of their estimated original ridge height. In a randomized clinical trial,[6] 90 edentulous patients were assigned to three different treatment modalities: (1) new complete dentures only; (2) new complete dentures with a mandibular vestibu-

loplasty; and (3) new dentures with implant support. Patients were followed for 5 years to assess various functional improvements. Altogether, no obvious differences were found between the two groups with conventional dentures, but the group with implant-supported overdentures demonstrated significant functional improvement and expressed higher treatment satisfaction.

Aging and Implant-Supported Overdentures

Overdentures supported by two intraforaminal implants is a well-established treatment modality and its effectiveness is demonstrated in many reports.[2,7] The following principles have been established for treatment with overdentures:

1. Placement of two intraforaminal implants is sufficient for denture stabilization.
2. Ball anchors or a splinting bar are recommended for denture anchorage.
3. Risks and patient morbidity can be minimized with a short one-stage surgical procedure.
4. Most elderly edentulous patients who can undergo a short surgical intervention despite various systemic problems are viable candidates.

Such treatment criteria sparked debate on the local, systemic, and behavioral aspects of aging and the risks of osseointegration in poor-quality bone encountered in older patients. Various systemic factors were considered to be contraindications as related to the surgical procedures or to the process and maintenance of osseointegration itself. Bone quality and quantity were often regarded to be insufficient in elderly patients. Furthermore, it was assumed that patient compliance, maintenance

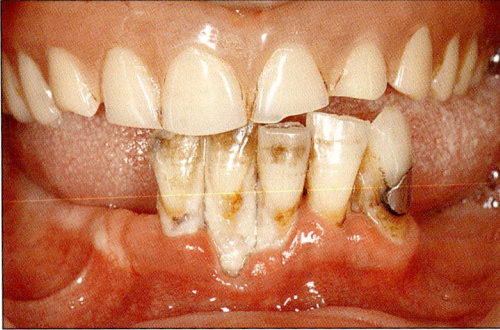

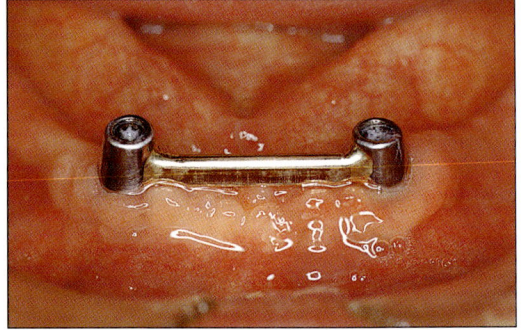

Figs 10-4a and 10-4b This patient was motivated to perform good oral hygiene after receiving implants. *(left)* Residual mandibular dentition and old maxillary complete denture prior to treatment. *(right)* Hygiene improved after placement of two implants connected with a bar.

of good oral hygiene, and participation in the recall program would not be consistent. However, placement of implants may make patients more aware of oral problems and motivate them to care for their oral health (Figs 10-4a and 10-4b). Therefore, an individual risk assessment for each patient is more important than establishment of strict exclusion criteria.

Systemic osteoporosis is often considered to negatively impact osseointegration in elderly patients, but numerous studies point to the contrary. Bone conditions have been found to vary within individuals,[8] and this may also be true for the arch that exhibits site-specific characteristics. Comparative evaluation of jawbone behavior related to age and site specificity indicate that implant therapy in older patients may be highly successful. Thus, it may be favorable to extract hopeless teeth and place implants as long as sufficient bone quantity is available. Postponement of treatment may result in more advanced atrophy, which can lead to additional problems as patients age and as their systemic health deteriorates (Figs 10-5a to 10-5g).

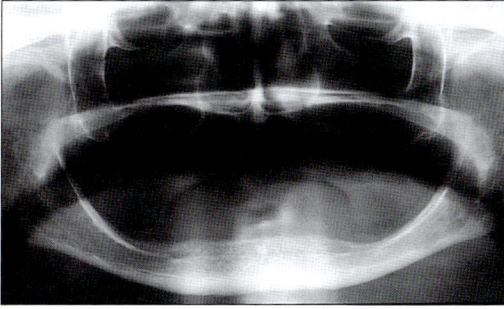

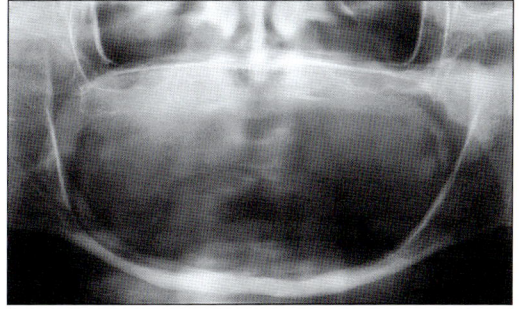

Figs 10-5a and 10-5b Progression of atrophy in one patient over a 15-year period. The patient was denied implant treatment 15 years ago due to advanced age *(left)*. The patient is no longer able to wear the mandibular complete denture *(right)*.

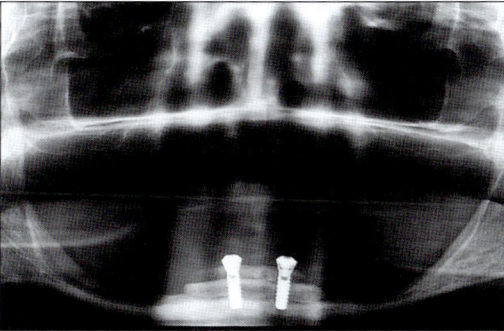

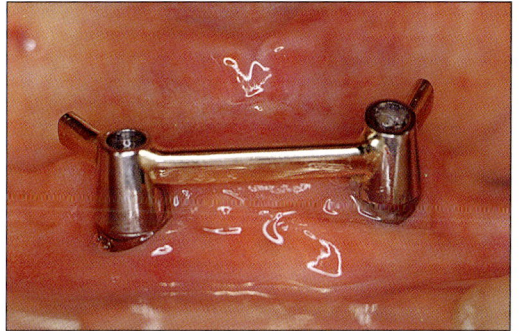

Figs 10-5c and 10-5d The patient received implants in combination with a bone graft. Bone augmentation could have been avoided if the patient had been treated 15 years ago.

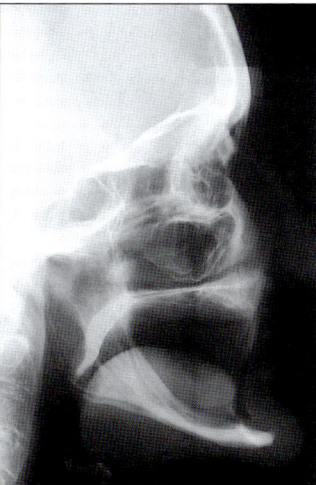

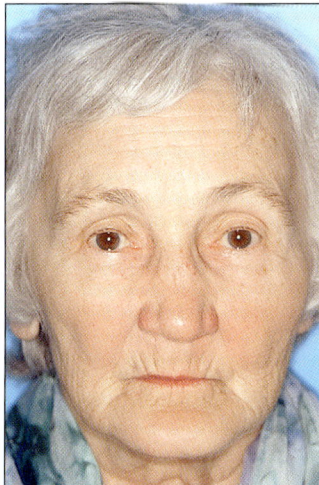

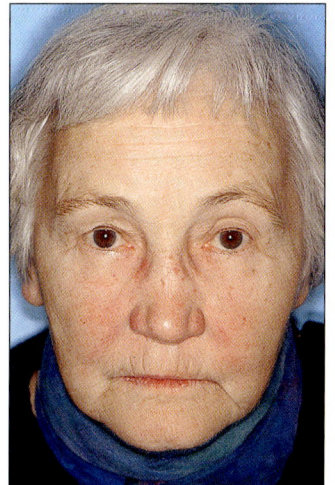

Figs 10-5e and 10-5f Appearance before treatment.

Fig 10-5g Appearance after treatment with implant-supported dentures.

Patients who benefit from mandibular overdentures

- Are usually elderly (65 to 80+ years)
- Are edentulous in the maxilla and mandible
- Have worn complete dentures for many years
- Are uncomfortable with a complete mandibular denture
- Demand stabilization of denture
- If not yet edentulous, they exhibit extremely reduced residual dentition that cannot be maintained

Patients who benefit from maxillary overdentures

- Are in the younger segment of older patients (50 to 60 years)
- Have no experience with maxillary removable prosthesis
- Exhibit hopeless residual maxillary dentition
- Are fearful of becoming edentulous
- Have high esthetic demands
- Have natural teeth or fixed prosthesis in mandible
- Desire fixed reconstruction

Clinical Considerations for Overdenture Therapy

Indications for Overdentures and Prosthesis Design

There are two types of patients who may benefit from overdenture treatment[9]: completely edentulous elderly patients who desire stabilization of the mandibular denture and patients with an edentulous maxilla who request fixed prostheses first (see box).

Many clinicians tend to believe that fixed prostheses with multiple implants are optimal and select the type of prosthesis according to the number of implants that can be placed in the edentulous arch. However, as dental medicine becomes increasingly evidence based, consideration of specific decision-making criteria becomes important. These criteria include fabrication techniques, biomechanics, biology, and patient-related factors, such as ease of handling, esthetics, cost, and treatment invasiveness.

Certain principles can be followed to address the technical and biologic aspects of overdenture fabrication.

Guidelines for Mandibular Overdenture Fabrication

Two intraforaminal implants of standard size (approximately 4 mm in diameter and a minimum of 8 mm in length) are recommended. The distance between the implants should be 15 to 25 mm, depending on the size and curvature of the anterior arch. The implants can be splinted with a clip-bar (resilient retention) or a U-shaped bar (rigid retention) as well as single anchors, such ball attachments. Three or four implants are recommended when implants of reduced length or diameter are used.

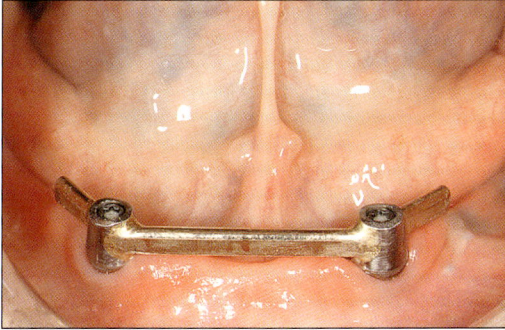

Fig 10-6a Two intraforaminal implants connected with a bar.

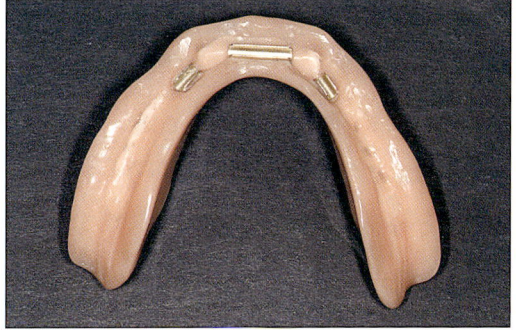

Fig 10-6b Inner surface of mandibular denture with bar retainers fixed in resin denture material.

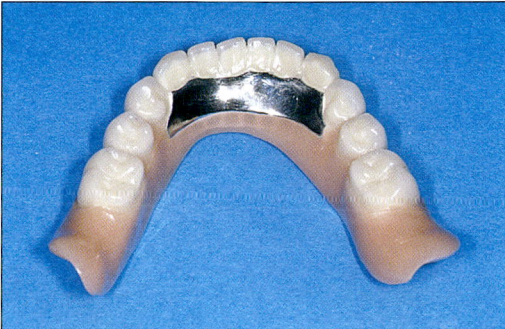

Fig 10-6c Denture reinforced with a cast metal framework to avoid fractures.

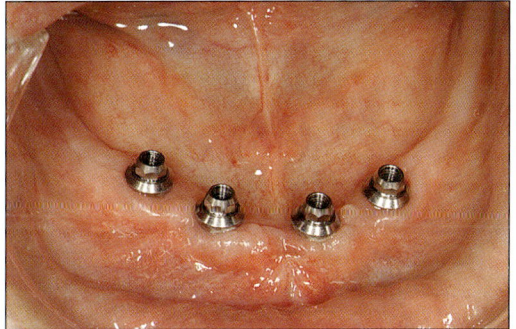

Fig 10-7 Four intraforaminal implants in close position. Bar segments may be too short. A fixed cantilever prosthesis can be mounted.

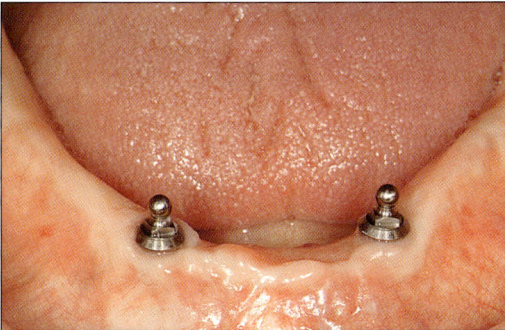

Fig 10-8a Two intraforaminal implants connected with single ball anchors.

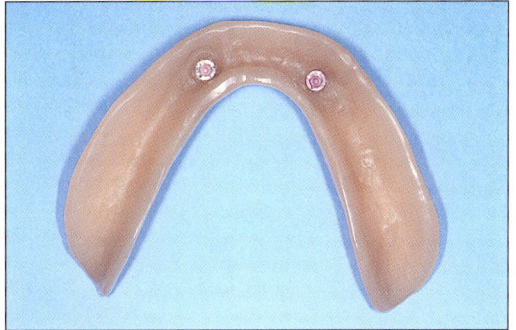

Fig 10-8b Inner surface with retainer for ball anchors.

In this case, the distance between the implants should be 12 to 15 mm to allow for a reasonable length of the bar segments. If four or more implants are placed, a fixed cantilever prosthesis is recommended (Figs 10-6 to 10-8).

Guidelines for Maxillary Overdenture Fabrication

A minimum of four implants evenly distributed over the anterior arch is preferred. Standard size and reduced-diameter implants can be used in the same arch. A splinting bar (preferably rigid) is recommended, although ball anchors can be used for temporary adaptation. Retention with ball anchors may not be adequate in every situation due to divergent implant axes. It is suggested that the denture base be reinforced with a cast metal framework; this increases the initial cost, but it may reduce maintenance costs since fractures and other complications can be avoided (Figs 10-9a to 10-9f).

Special anatomic situations, such as congenital defects, require individual fabrication of maxillary prostheses (Figs 10-10a to 10-10e). Ball anchors can be used in combination with remaining tooth roots for overdenture anchorage. Such treatment concepts are empirical in part, but clinical evidence will be obtained from short- and long-term observations.

Biomechanical Considerations

Various studies have analyzed the biomechanical aspects of overdentures (primarily mandibular overdentures) by means of experimental laboratory methods, such as finite element analysis, or clinical measurements. There is much debate over the type of retention that should be used with overdentures: Should the denture be supported by implants or tissue? Should rigid or resilient retention devices be used? How many implants and retention devices are ideal? Are splinted or unsplinted devices better? Various hypotheses also exist, but many lack clinical relevance. One hypothesis suggested that the bar connecting the implants should be parallel to the hinge axis; this rule was followed by many clinicians, but no studies have supported this claim. One long-term study (5 to 15 years) analyzed the influence of placing the bar parallel to the hinge axis on peri-implant parameters, including the clinical attachment level.[10] The effect of the type of retention mechanism and device, ie, rigid versus resilient, splinted versus unsplinted, was also assessed. No significant correlations were found. Implant stability was high (> 95%), and only minor clinical attachment loss was measured around all implants.

In vitro stress analyses of splinted and unsplinted mandibular intraforaminal implants have revealed few differences. One in vivo study[11] suggested that ball anchors are preferred because they provide better load distribution on the posterior mandibular bone. A series of three-dimensional force measurements with two intraforaminal ITI implants (Straumann, Waldenburg, Switzerland) in completely edentulous patients revealed no significant differences when different attachment devices and retention mechanisms were compared.[12,13] Axial forces were dominant but always accompanied by transverse forces. These results were confirmed by other investigations that tested Brånemark implants (Nobel Biocare, Göteborg, Sweden) with another measuring equipment.[14] When distal extensions were used, the splinting effect disappeared, ie, the same force patterns were observed as with unsplinted implants.

One may wonder whether distal extensions are necessary or if they will break. In fact, distal extensions provide a high level of stability against lateral forces, particularly in the mandible, and may protect the vulnerable denture-bearing tissue from loading forces. They should not extend beyond the position of the first premolar of the mandibular prosthesis, and they cannot compensate for a short central segment.

Figs 10-9a to 10-9f Construction of a four-implant, bar-retained maxillary overdenture with a horseshoe design.

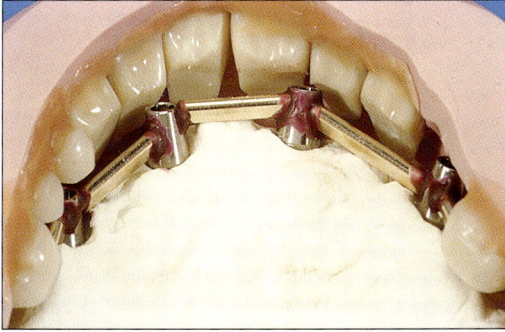

Fig 10-9a The close position of the bar and anterior teeth provides optimum denture stability when the patient bites with the anterior teeth.

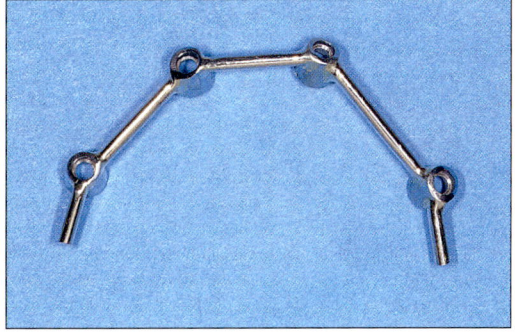

Fig 10-9b Completed bar.

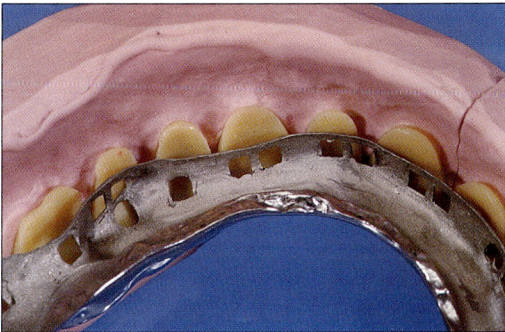

Fig 10-9c Individual cast metal framework provides optimum stability of the overdenture.

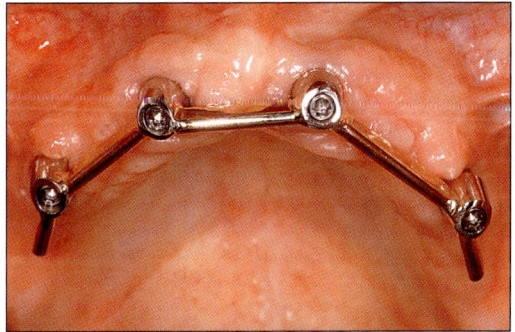

Fig 10-9d Bar in situ.

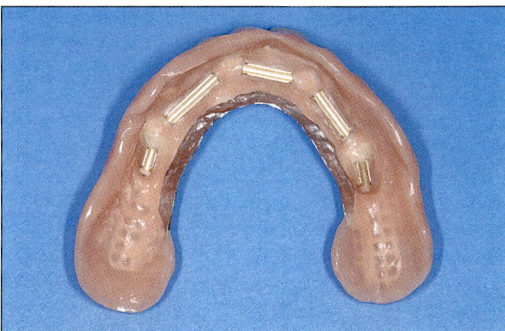

Fig 10-9e Inner surface of the maxillary overdenture showing bar retainers fixed in denture resin base material.

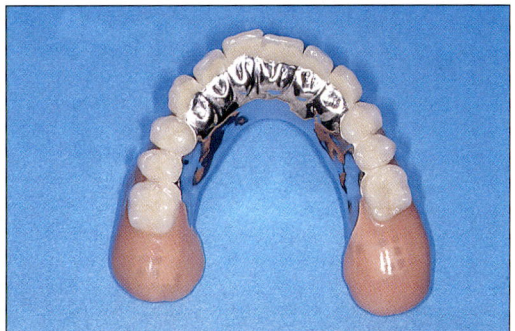

Fig 10-9f Horseshoe prosthesis design with open palate. The cast metal framework allows for an elegant, slim design of the overdenture.

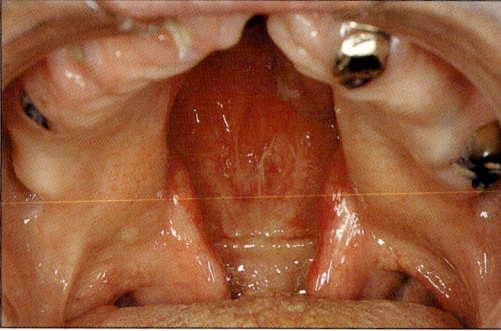

Fig 10-10a A 90-year-old patient with a cleft palate and loss of remaining roots that were used for anchorage of a maxillary complete denture.

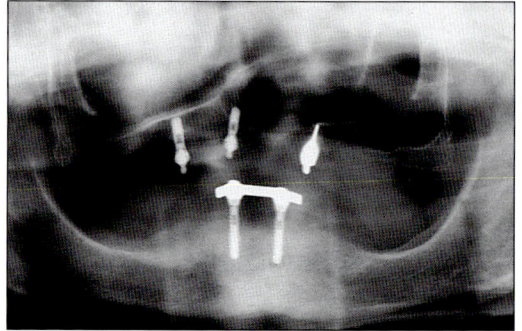

Fig 10-10b Treatment included placement of two maxillary implants on the right and two mandibular intraforaminal implants. One maxillary left root coping was restored.

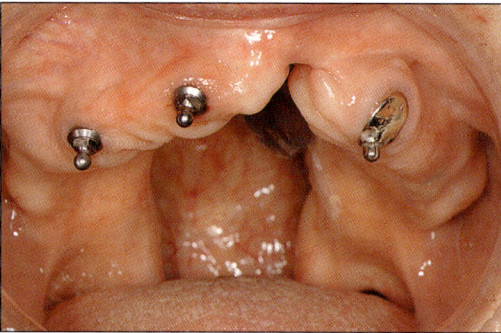

Fig 10-10c Intraoral view of the maxilla after placement of implants with ball anchors.

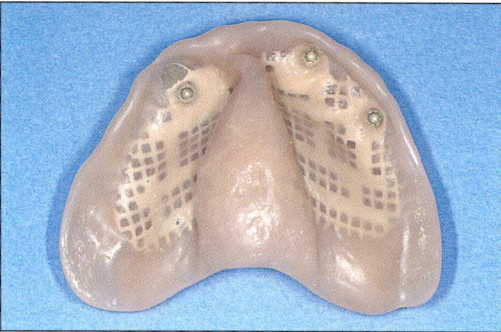

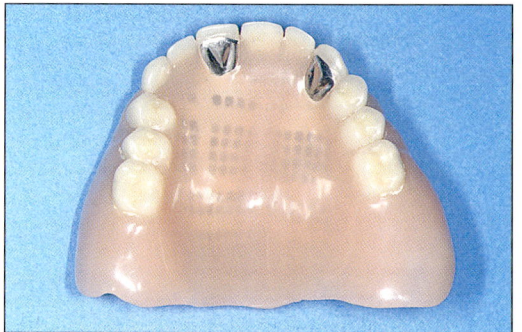

Figs 10-10d and 10-10e A complete denture design with full palatal coverage and obturator was necessary. The metal framework embedded in the resin base material is slightly visible.

Among the large body of studies on mandibular overdentures, no evidence supports the superiority of one attachment device or retention mechanism over another. (See chapter 11 for further discussion of attachment systems.)

Less information is available for retention of maxillary overdentures. While use of a bar with a rigid denture connection is commonly preferred,[9] others suggest a bar with a resilient connection.[15] However, there is no scientific evidence to support this method. A pilot study compared repeated in vivo measurements of maxillary implants supporting either a fixed denture or an overdenture with a rigid bar connection.[16] Similar force magnitudes and patterns were found, suggesting that a rigid bar with a connected overdenture performs in a manner similar to a fixed prosthesis under loading conditions. From experimental measurements, it was concluded that maxillary overdentures are best supported by multiple implants, connected by a rigid bar, and reinforced with a metal framework to enhance rigidity of the superstructure.[17]

Treatment Success with Overdentures

Implant Survival

Comparison of studies that discuss success, failure, and survival rates is difficult because parameters and indices are applied in different ways to determine short- and long-term implant stability. Most studies available on mandibular overdentures report a success rate of 90% to 100%. Neither the number of supporting implants nor the type of retention device has been found to affect the rate of survival. The mandibular overdenture is reported to be superior to conventional dentures.[18]

In contrast, results of implants placed in the edentulous maxilla, particularly in conjunction with overdentures, are less favorable. Various studies have shown a surprisingly high early failure rate for implants placed in the edentulous maxilla.[19] Furthermore, minor bone resorption surrounding the cervical portion of the implants may be evident. Some patients in the same study[18,19] lost the majority or all of their implants. If a distinction between the degree of atrophy in the maxilla and the bone quality is made, results show that failures in the maxilla are related to short implants, poor bone quality, and a small number of implants. This combination of negative factors was often found when overdentures were placed in emergency situations. For well-planned maxillary overdenture cases, there is a higher survival rate compared to conventional dentures, healthy marginal soft tissues, and stable marginal bone found around implants with normal bone conditions. However, for some patients, ongoing bone resorption can be observed. Although bone grafting is often suggested for patients with advanced atrophy, this surgical procedure typically results in a high percentage of implant losses and increased bone resorption.

Prosthetic Results

Assessment of prosthetic results can be challenging, since a clear distinction of normal maintenance, repairs, and adjustment of prostheses is not made. Maintenance due to normal wear can become excessive, and discriminatory criteria for assessment of service, complications, and repairs are needed. Such a differentiation is, in part, a quantitative one. Parameters to assess specific aspects of prosthetic reconstruction are not well defined, are not generally accepted, and may vary among studies. Complications can vary widely from a simple adjustment to a remake of the entire prosthesis. Proposals for classification of prosthetic service have been made.[20–22]

Clinically, the overdenture is simpler and its initial treatment is less costly than that for fixed prostheses. However, the overdenture has more single components (abutments, clips, bars, anchors, and female retainers) that can create complications and require service. It has been proposed to measure the time required for service and repairs or to count the number of visits by the patient to the clinician as a reliable measure for comparisons. A 5-year longitudinal study[22] comparing two resilient retention mechanisms found more complications with bars than with ball attachments. Another study compared complications with rigid and resilient retention mechanisms for mandibular overdentures supported by two implants during a time period from 5 to 15 years. The incidence of all types of complications did not differ significantly between the two groups. However, replacement of the entire retention mechanism was more frequent with ball anchors and round clip-bars (ie, resilient mechanisms) than with rigid bars.[23] Another study demonstrated a high probability that some adjustment would be necessary with maxillary overdentures, particularly in the first year after delivery of the dentures.[21] However, these adjustments were mostly related to sore spots caused by the denture base or retightening of the bar screws. The first problem is also typical with conventional dentures and is easily resolved.

Patient-Related Factors

Treatment outcomes should not consider solely implant and prosthesis survival, but should also consider the physiologic and psychologic impacts of overdenture treatment. Treatment outcome must be measured by self-assessment using questionnaires to evaluate quality of life. In fact, clinical experience suggests that patients' response to implant therapy parallels a significant improvement in quality of life. From an economic point of view, overdentures supported by two to four implants may be preferred over fixed prostheses because costs are reduced. Esthetic appearance, facial morphology, and restitution of lost hard and soft tissues may be provided more easily, if not better, with overdentures than with fixed prostheses.

Controlled clinical trials and cross-over studies compared the use of different overdenture support with fixed prostheses.[24,25] The investigations included subjective and objective parameters, functional assessment, and overall patient satisfaction. Patient preferences also were considered to have a potential impact on the design and interpretation of clinical trials. Comparisons made using randomized clinical trials of patient expectations before and after treatment with complete dentures and implant-supported dentures demonstrated higher overall patient satisfaction with overdentures.

Summary

Mandibular overdentures with a few supporting intraforaminal implants are a predictable and successful treatment modality. Two implants will mostly serve the purpose. In the case of advanced atrophy and short implants (< 8 mm) three implants are recommended.

There is no evidence for the superiority of one retention device and mechanism. Thus, the system for denture connection to the intraforaminal implants can be selected according to the specific clinical situation and individual needs of the patient.

Maxillary overdentures have become better documented in the last few years, and prosthetic concepts and treatment protocols have been established. There is still a great need for long-term surveys to analyze treatment outcomes with planned cases. As long as comparative data of planned maxillary overdentures are lacking, a minimum of four implants with a rigidly splinting bar must be recommended as the standard of care.

References

1. Brånemark P-I, Zarb GA, Albrektsson T. Tissue-Integrated Prostheses. Chicago: Quintessence, 1985.

2. Mericske-Stern R. Clinical evaluation of overdenture restorations supported by osseointegrated titanium implants. A retrospective study. Int J Oral Maxillofac Implants 1990;5:375–383.

3. Buser D, Mericske-Stern R, Bernard JP, et al. Long-term evaluation of non-submerged ITI implants. Part 1: 8-year life table analysis of a prospective multicenter study with 2,359 implants. Clin Oral Implants Res 1997;8:161–172.

4. Makkonen TA, Holmberg S, Niemi L, Olsson C, Tammisalo T, Peltola J. A 5-year prospective clinical study of Astra Tech dental implants supporting fixed bridges or overdentures in the edentulous mandible. Clin Oral Implants Res 1997;8:469–475.

5. Närhi TO, Ettinger RL, Lam EW. Radiographic findings, ridge resorption, and subjective complaints of complete denture patients. Int J Prosthodont 1997;10:183–189.

6. Raghoebar GM, Meijer HJA, Stegenga B, van't Hof MA, van Oort RP, Vissink A. Effectiveness of three treatment modalities for the edentulous mandible. Clin Oral Implants Res 2000;11:195–201.

7. Mericske-Stern R, Zarb GA. Overdentures: An alternative implant methodology for edentulous patients. Int J Prosthodont 1993;6:203–208.

8. Frost HM. Changing views about "Osteoporoses" (a 1998 overview). Osteoporos Int 1999;10:345–352.

9. Mericske-Stern R. Treatment outcomes with implant-supported overdentures. Clinical considerations. J Prosthet Dent 1998;79:66–73.

10. Oetterli M, Kiener P, Mericske-Stern R. A longitudinal study on mandibular implants supporting an overdenture: The influence of retention mechanism and anatomic-prosthetic variables on peri-implant parameters. Int J Prosthodont 2001;14:536–542.

11. Menicucci G, Lorenzetti M, Pera P, Preti G. Mandibular implant-retained overdenture: Finite element analysis of two anchorage systems. Int J Oral Maxillofac Implants 1998;13:369–376.

12. Mericske-Stern R, Piotti M, Sirtes G. 3-D in vivo force measurements on mandibular implants supporting overdentures. A comparative study. Clin Oral Implants Res 1996;7:387–396.

13. Mericske-Stern R. Three-dimensional force measurements with mandibular overdentures connected to implants by ball-shaped retentive anchors. A clinical study. Int J Oral Maxillofac Implants 1998;13:36–43.

14. Duyck J, Van Oosterwyck H, Vander Sloten J, De Cooman M, Puers R, Naert I. In vivo forces on oral implants supporting a mandibular overdenture: The influence of attachment system. Clin Oral Investig 1999; 99:201–207.

15. Naert I, Gizani S, van Steenberghe D. Rigidly splinted implants in the resorbed maxilla to retain a hinging overdenture: A series of clinical reports for up to 4 years. J Prosthet Dent 1998;79:156–164.

16. Mericske-Stern R, Venetz E, Fahrländer F, Bürgin W. In vivo force measurements on maxillary implants supporting a fixed prosthesis or an overdenture: A pilot study. J Prosthet Dent 2000;84:535–547.

17. Glantz PO, Nilner K. Biomechanical aspects on overdenture treatment. J Dent 1997;25(suppl 1):21–24.

18. Carr AB. Successful long-term treatment outcomes in the field of osseointegrated implants: Prosthodontic determinants. Int J Prosthodont 1998;11:502–512.

19. Chan MF, Närhi TO, de Baat C, Kalk W. Treatment of the atrophic edentulous maxilla with implant-supported overdentures. A review of the literature. Int J Prosthodont 1998;11:207–215.

20. Payne AGT, Solomons YF. The prosthodontic maintenance requirements of mandibular mucosa- and implant-supported overdentures: A review of the literature. Int J Prosthodont 2000;13:238–245.

21. Kiener P, Oetterli M, Mericske E, Mericske-Stern R. Effectiveness of maxillary overdentures supported by implants: Maintenance and prosthetic complications. Int J Prosthodont 2001;14:133–140.

22. Gotfredsen K, Holm B. Implant-supported mandibular overdentures retained with ball or bar attachments: A randomized prospective 5-year study. Int J Prosthodont 2000;13:125–130.

23. Dudic A, Mericske-Stern R. Retention mechanisms and prosthetic complications of implant-supported mandibular overdentures: Long-term results. Clin Implant Dent Relat Res 2002;4:212–219.

24. Tang L, Lund JP, Tache R, Clokie CM, Feine JS. A within-subject comparison of mandibular long-bar and hybrid implant-supported prostheses: Psychometric evaluation and patient preference. J Dent Res 1997;76:1675–1683.

25. Feine JS, Awad MA, Lund JP. The impact of patient preference on the design and interpretation of clinical trials. Community Dent Oral Epidemiol 1998;26: 70–74.

CHAPTER 11

The Influence of Attachment Systems on Implant-Retained Mandibular Overdentures

Ignace Naert

Replacement of lost tissues with complete dentures is challenging for both dentist and patient.[1,2] However, the efficacy of some endosseous implant systems now allows patients to be successfully treated with implant-retained overdentures. Several studies report the clear benefits of overdenture treatment compared to conventional dentures for a number of aspects, including esthetics, speech, chewing, fit and retention, function, and quality of life.[3,4]

A variety of attachment systems have been used to retain overdentures. Generally, these can be classified as clips-and-bars, balls, magnets, and telescopic copings (rigid or nonrigid). The selection of an attachment system is mainly related to the personal choice of the practitioner and/or laboratory responsible, based on experience and training.

Advanced alveolar bone resorption may favor a connector that offers a considerable amount of horizontal stability, such as bars or telescopic attachments.[5] When alveolar resorption is minimal, magnets offer an alternative solution, although they provide the least retention force compared to the other attachments and lose their initial retention capacity rather soon.[6] Balls are ideal for patients with a narrow jaw anatomy, because bars leave insufficient tongue space.[7] Although nonrigid telescopic copings produce low stress at the implants and surrounding bone, as do ball or magnet attachments, rigid telescopic copings induce considerably higher stresses. The concern here is not the biologic response to these stresses (potential marginal bone resorption) but the increased risk for implant fatigue and eventual fracture of the implant or its components.[8] On the other hand, the more rigid the connector, the least loading on the edentulous posterior areas and, indirectly, the least alveolar bone resorption.

Cost is an important factor to consider as well, especially in this kind of treatment. Magnets and balls are the least expensive; bars and especially telescopic copings are the most expensive.

Very few studies have prospectively compared clinical outcomes.[9–13] The clinical trial discussed in this chapter investigated the treatment outcome of splinted (bars) and unsplinted (balls and magnets) implants retaining a mandibular hinging overdenture 5 and 10 years after delivery of the prosthesis. Telescopic copings, due their limited application, are out of scope here.

Clinical Trial

Thirty-six completely edentulous patients with a mean age of 63 years were enrolled in the study.[6,14] All patients had complaints about their existing dentures, even after technical improvement. The exclusion criteria for patient selection were insufficient bone volume to harbor at least two 10-mm implants, retrognathic mandible, psychologic difficulties accepting a removable denture, gagging reflex, less than 1 year of edentulism in the mandible, absence of a maxillary complete denture, and administrative or physical considerations that would seriously affect the surgical procedure or hinder a 5-year follow-up. All patients were recalled 10 years after delivery as well.

Each patient was provided with two screw-shaped commercially pure titanium implants (Brånemark system, Nobel Biocare, Göteborg, Sweden) in the symphyseal area of the mandible.[15] Overall, 73 implants were placed and transmucosally connected to the abutments 3 to 5 months later.

The 36 patients were randomly allocated into one of the three groups, each with a different attachment system (Figs 11-1a to 11-1c). The bar group, considered the reference group, was provided with an egg-shaped Dolder bar (Cendres et Metaux SA, Biel, Switzerland) splinting the two implants. The magnet group used two open-field magnets

(Dyna Engineering BV, Bergen op Zoom, The Netherlands) as attachment system. In the ball group, overdentures were retained by two ball attachments with rubber rings (SDCB 115-17, Nobel Biocare, Göteborg, Sweden). The occlusion was set in centric relation without anterior tooth contact. The lateral excursion and protrusion were assessed on an articulator and intraorally to secure a balanced articulation.

Patients were scheduled for follow-up visits 1 week after prosthesis insertion and 4, 6, 12, 24, 36, 48, 60, and 120 months after abutment installation. The results at 10 years after delivery concern implant and marginal bone outcome only; all other data refer to the 5-year recall visits.[14]

Each follow-up visit included evaluation of the presence or absence of plaque and mucosal bleeding (defined as bleeding elicited 20 seconds after running a periodontal probe 1 mm into the mucosal sulcus parallel to the abutment wall). The minimum and maximum scores per abutment were 0 and 4, respectively.

The pocket probing depth (PD) and gingival recession were measured with a periodontal probe at six sites around each abutment. The rigidity of the implant-bone continuum was evaluated by means of the Periotest device (Siemens, Bensheim, Germany) from –8 (very stable) to +50 (very mobile).

An implant was considered a failure if: (1) a peri-implant radiolucency could be detected, (2) the slightest sign of mobility (Periotest value > +5) was detected, and (3) signs or symptoms such as pain or infection were reported. Marginal bone level, measured radiographically by the same independent investigator, was rated mesially and distally using a long-cone apparatus.

Overdenture retention was measured by means of a dynamometer with a maximum capacity of 20 N; the mean of three repeated measurements was calculated.[12] The mechanical complications of the attachment compo-

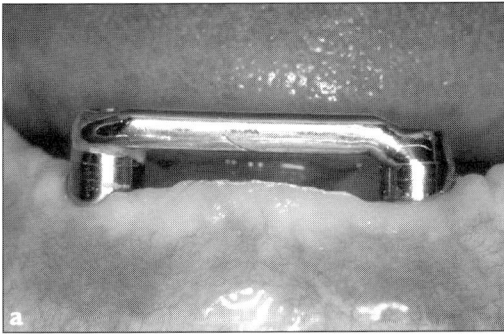

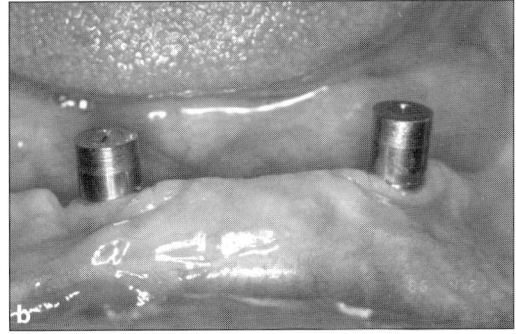

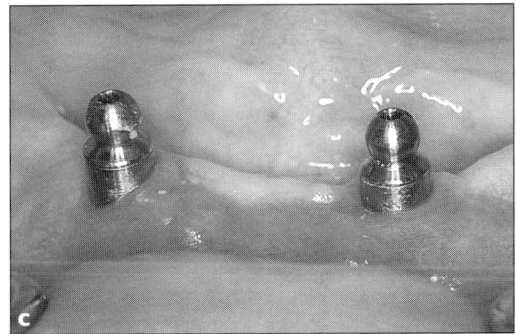

Figs 11-1a to 11-1c Three different attachment systems: (*a*) bar, (*b*) magnet, and (*c*) ball.

nents were recorded in addition to the soft tissue complications of the denture-bearing area (mucositis, soreness, ulcer decubitus, and hyperplasia) for the entire observation period.

Patient satisfaction was investigated through a questionnaire. Patients answered questions on a scale ranging from 1 (very bad) to 9 (very good). A second part included questions with a "yes/no" response.

Function of the temporomandibular joints and masticatory muscles was assessed according to an anamnestic and clinical dysfunction index.[16]

To avoid a clustering effect, the mean scores of the two implants per patient were considered. Differences of presence or absence of plaque, mucosal bleeding, Periotest values, marginal bone, and attachment level per group, as well as over time, were analyzed by a modified analysis of variance test. For the analysis of marginal bone changes, the intraexaminer's variability (0.2 mm) was set as the detection threshold for marginal bone changes. Differences in patient satisfaction per group at year 5, as well as the variations in patient satisfaction over time, were analyzed by a nonparametric Kruskal-Wallis analysis of variance test. Both the objective and subjective retention of the overdentures, for all three groups, was analyzed by a nonparametric Spearman correlation analysis. The level of significance was set at .05 unless otherwise stated.

Table 11-1 Frequency distribution of denture-supporting mucosa complications and the corresponding number of patients who experienced the complications during the 5-year follow-up per group

	Bar		Magnet		Ball	
Complication	No. of occurrences	No. of patients	No. of occurrences	No. of patients	No. of occurrences	No. of patients
Mucositis	12	5	2	2	3	3
Soreness	3	2	0	0	0	0
Ulcer decubitis	6	3	12	4	8	6
Hyperplasia	9	7	4	3	3	3

Data used with permission from Naert et al.[6,14]

Patient Follow-up and Implant Failure

Five patients did not return for the 5-year follow-up. One patient, from the magnet group, was dissatisfied with the prosthetic treatment outcome. Four years after treatment, she had a new overdenture made on a bar by a private practitioner. Ten years after delivery, 10 patients had died.

During the 10-year period, none of the loaded implants failed. Only one implant had failed at the time of abutment surgery (due to mobility) and was replaced in the same session by a new implant that healed uneventfully.

Peri-implant Outcome and Bone Changes

At year 5, the magnet group harbored the most plaque. It is unknown whether the magnetic field influences this accumulation. Retention problems and prosthetic complications with the magnet systems may account for a lack of compliance with the prescribed oral hygiene regimen.[17] The ball attachments harbored the least amount of plaque. This can be explained by the free-standing implants, which perhaps allows for easier oral hygiene by the patient.

Mucositis and hyperplasia occurred more often in the bar group, while ulcer decubitus was observed more often in the magnet and ball groups (Table 11-1). Mucositis and ulcer decubitus continued to be present in the same patients throughout the 5 years of the study, while hyperplasia was observed in increasing numbers of patients over time. These findings apply to all three treatment groups. However, the plaque index, as well as mucosal bleeding at year 5 did not significantly differ from the outcome at year 1.[18]

No mucosal bleeding of the soft tissues around the abutments was found in any group at year 5. Furthermore, for all groups, no significant correlation was found between mucosal bleeding on probing and total bone loss during

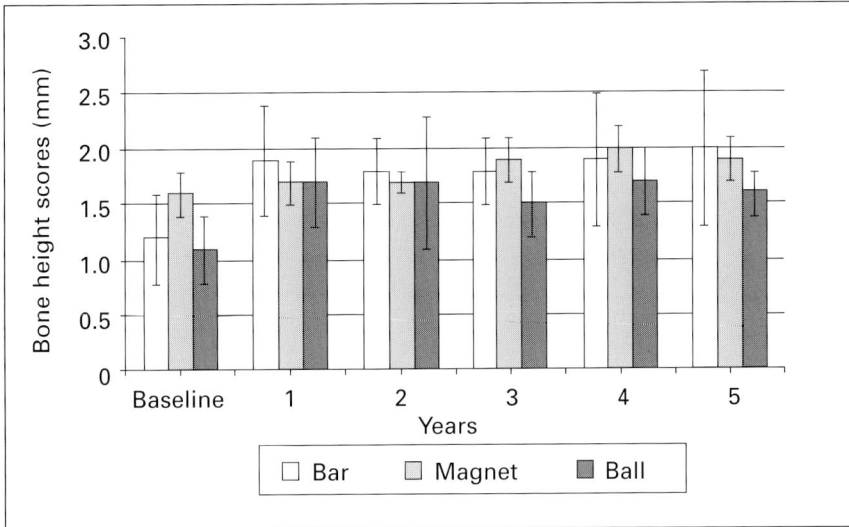

Fig 11-2 Mean (SD) marginal bone level from baseline (abutment connection) to year 5 for each group. The reference is the implant-abutment junction. (Data used with permission from Naert et al.[6,14])

the 5-year period. This finding is in agreement with other research.[19–22] No difference in attachment level could be found among the three groups 1,[9] 5,[14] or 10 years after treatment.

The mean difference between the marginal bone level and the probing attachment level at year 5 was 1 mm, which corroborates the observations of Quirynen et al.[23]

No statistical differences were found among the three groups for marginal bone loss scores between years 1 and 5, nor between baseline (abutment connection) and year 5 (Fig 11-2). This corroborates results from Gotfredsen and Holm[13] for Astra Tech implants supporting ball- or bar-attached overdentures after a period of

5 years. In the present study, the mean bone loss between baseline and year 1 was 0.59 mm for the bar group, 0.27 mm for the magnet group, and 0.55 mm for the ball group. The annual marginal bone changes, the first year excluded (−0.03 mm for the bar group, −0.05 mm for the magnet group, and 0.01 mm for the ball group) showed no between-group differences. Mean marginal bone loss between baseline and year 5 was at most 1.0 mm for 87% of the implants (Table 11-2). Figure 11-3 illustrates the small changes from baseline up to year 10.

For all groups, the Periotest values at year 5 were significantly lower compared to year 1

Table 11-2 Categorical distribution of mean marginal bone loss between baseline (abutment connection) and year 5

Mean marginal bone loss (mm)	No. of implants
−0.3–0	9
0.1 –0.5	27
0.6– 1.0	17
1.1 –2.0	8
2.1 –3.0	1

Data used with permission from Naert et al.[6,14]

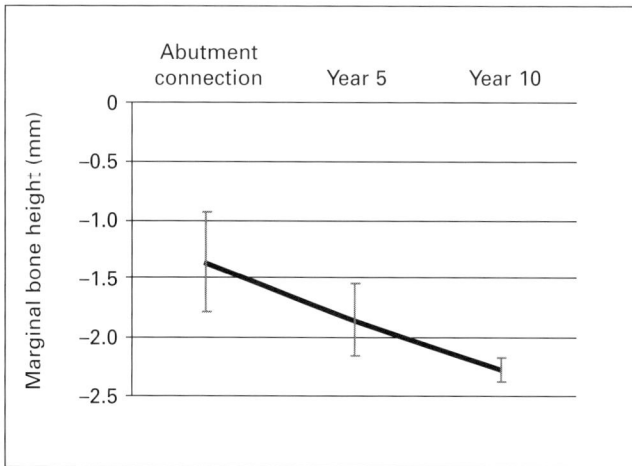

Fig 11-3 Mean (SD) marginal bone level from baseline (abutment connection) to year 10 for all three groups. The reference is the implant-abutment junction.

(P = .003) (Fig 11-4). The total mean Periotest values decreased between baseline and year 5 for bars (1.6 units), magnets (0.7 units), and balls (2 units). The magnet group presented the smallest total Periotest value changes over the 5-year period, revealing it to be the least strain-provoking system. From a finite element analysis,[24] it was concluded that implants should be unsplinted when overdentures are used in order to reduce stress.

Prosthetic Retention

At year 5, the highest retention force was measured in the bar group (1240 g; range, 0 to 2000 g), and the lowest force was measured in the magnet group (110 g; range, 0 to 456 g) (Table 11-3). This finding is in agreement with results at 3 years postdelivery[12] and previous reports.[4,25–30] Comparison of the retention forces between baseline (prosthesis installa-

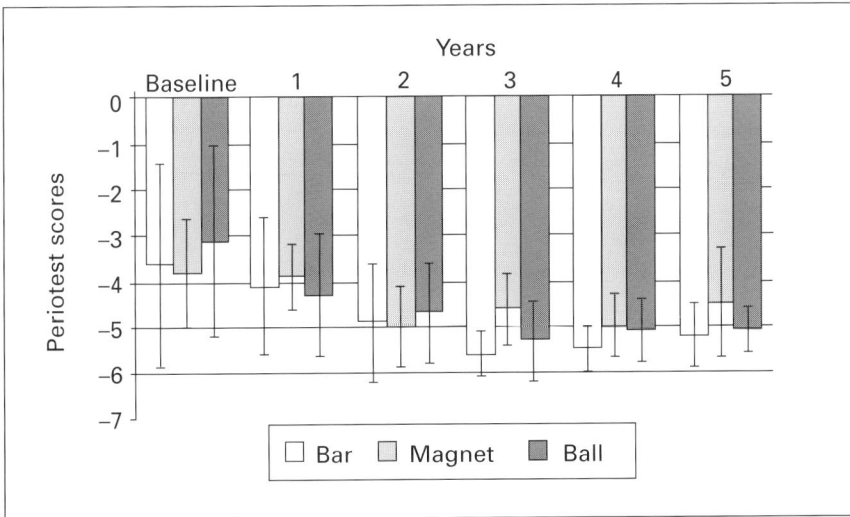

Fig 11-4 Mean (SD) Periotest values from baseline (abutment connection) to year 5 for each group. (Data used with permission from Naert et al.[6,14])

Table 11-3 Mean retention force (in grams, mean of three repeated measurements) of overdentures measured by a dynamometer

	Bar	Magnet	Ball
Baseline (delivery of prosthesis)	1677	370	655
Force, year 1	1855	362	730
Force, year 5	1240	110	567
Relative decrease from baseline to year 5	44%	70%	33%

Data used with permission from Naert et al.[6,14]

tion) and year 5 revealed a decrease of retention over time for all three groups. The magnet group lost, on average, 70% of its retention force over time, while the ball group lost only 33%. Loss of force in the bar group can be ex-plained by deactivation of the clip-bar components because reactivation took place only at the patient's request. Magnet and ball attachments were renewed rather than reactivated.

Table 11-4 Frequency distribution of prosthetic complications for the 5-year observation period per group

Prosthetic complication	Bars	Magnets*	Balls*
Retention element			
Wear	3	21	12
Corrosion	N/A	21	0
Fracture	N/A	1	11
Loosening of abutment screw	0	10	25
Loosening of gold screw	3	2	N/A
Clip activation	12	N/A	N/A
Clip change	3	N/A	N/A
Exchange of			
Rubber ring	N/A	N/A	13
O-box	N/A	N/A	16
Magnet	N/A	53	N/A
Rebasing	1	3	4
Remounting	0	1	0
New denture made	1	0	6

Data used with permission from Naert et al.[6,14]

*In the magnet and ball groups, each patient had two attachments.

Prosthetic Complications

The magnet and ball groups presented the highest incidence of prosthetic complications in comparison to the bar group. This is in accordance with some material,[9,31] but contradicts results from Gotfredsen and Holm.[13] For example, in the magnet group, frequent renewal of magnets was needed because of wear and corrosion. For the ball group, frequent tightening of the abutment screws and renewal of the O-rings and the O-ring housings were most commonly needed. The common complications for each of the three groups are summarized in Table 11-4. Bars presented the least number of prosthetic complications.[5,28] When comparing the 3-year[12] to the 5-year results,[6] the number of prosthetic complications for the unsplinted implant groups increased considerably during the last 2 years. This finding is in contrast to the results of Davis et al[2] and Gotfredsen and Holm,[13] in which the majority of complications appeared during the first year.

Table 11-5 Mean (SD) scores for patient satisfaction at baseline (delivery of prosthesis) and year 5*

	Bars		Magnets		Balls	
	Baseline	**Year 5**	**Baseline**	**Year 5**	**Baseline**	**Year 5**
How do you like your prosthesis in general?	8.3 (0.5)	8.7 (0.4)	7.3 (1.1)	6.6[†] (2.2)	7.9 (1.8)	7.4 (1.8)
How well does your new prosthesis remain in place?	8.6 (0.5)	8.0 (1.5)	8.0 (0.3)	6.3[†] (2.4)	8.2 (1.4)	8.9 (0.3)
How well can you eat with your new prosthesis?	8.6 (0.5)	8.7 (0.48)	7.8 (1.2)	6.4 (2.2)	8.4 (0.9)	8.5 (0.8)
How well can you talk with your new prosthesis?	8.6 (0.5)	7.8 (1.4)	8.5 (0.5)	7.3 (1.4)	8.5 (0.5)	8.6 (0.9)
How do you like the appearance of your new prosthesis?	8.5 (0.5)	8.2 (0.7)	8.5 (0.7)	7.7 (1.7)	6.7 (3.3)	7.7 (0.6)

Data used with permission from Naert et al.[6,14]

*Patients rated questions on a scale from 1 (very bad) to 9 (very good).

†Statistically different from the other groups at the 5% level.

Patient Satisfaction

Patient satisfaction for chewing comfort, phonetics, and esthetics in all groups varied little between baseline and year 5. However, prosthesis stability and chewing comfort scored significantly lower among patients in the magnet group than in other groups (*P* = .05) (Table 11-5). All patients said they would choose the same treatment again, even though the expectations of those in the magnet group were not met. This can be explained by the dramatic improvement in comparison to the patients' previous complete dentures.

In the study by Naert et al,[6] half of the patients, equally distributed among the groups, did not remove their dentures at night, even though they had been instructed to do so. Their refusal to remove their dentures underlines the psychosocial impact of edentulism.

Dysfunction

At the end of the observation period, only one patient in the magnet group reported anamnestic or clinical dysfunction, compared to nine patients who reported anamnestic or clinical dysfunction at the beginning of the study.

Summary

Overdentures supported by a few implants dramatically improve patient comfort and acceptance as well as oral function[32] compared to the conventional denture. Splinting the implants with a bar is not a prerequisite for the long-term survival or prognosis of implants in the mandible. In fact, magnets, balls, and bars have been found to exhibit similar peri-implant outcomes 5 years after treatment. Bars have been shown to provide the most retention force, while magnets provide the least, losing 70% of their force over time. Prosthetic complications are more common with magnets and balls, with magnet-retained overdentures requiring the most aftercare.

Acknowledgments

The author is indebted to Dr S. Gizani for her contribution to the reporting of 5-year data. The author also gratefully acknowledges Prof M. Quirynen and Prof D. van Steenberghe, of the Department of Periodontology, Catholic University Leuven, Belgium, for placing the implants and to Prof M. Vuylsteke, chair of the Department of Statistics, Computing Centre, Catholic University Leuven, for the statistical analysis.

This chapter is a summary of data published by Naert et al.[6,14]

References

1. Zarb G. Oral motor patterns and their relation to oral prostheses. J Prost Dent 1982;47:472–478.
2. Davis D. The role of implants in the treatment of edentulous patients. Int J Prosthodont 1990;3:42–50.
3. de Grandmont P, Feine JS, Taché R, et al. Within-subject comparisons of implant-supported mandibular prostheses: Psychometric evaluation. J Dent Res 1994;73:1096–1104.
4. Burns DR, Unger JW, Elswick RK Jr, Giglio JA. Prospective clinical evaluation of mandibular implant overdentures: Part II. Patient satisfaction and preference. J Prosthet Dent 1995;73:364–369.
5. Heckmann S, Farmand M, Wahl G. Erste erfahrungen mit Resilienzteleskopen bei der prothetetischen Versorgung enossaler Implantate. Zeitschrift Zahnärtzl Implantol 1993;9:188–193.
6. Naert I, Gizani S, Vuylsteke M, van Steenberghe D. A 5-year prospective randomized clinical trial on the influence of splinted and unsplinted oral implants in the mandibular overdenture therapy. Part II: Prosthetic aspects and patient satisfaction. J Oral Rehabil 1999;26:195–202.
7. Spiekermann H. Implantology. In: Rateitschak KH, Wolf HF (eds). Color Atlas of Dental Medicine. New York: Thieme Medical Publishers, 1995.
8. Heckmann SM, Winter W, Meyer M, Weber H, Wichmann MG. Overdenture attachment selection and the loading of implant and denture-bearing area. Part 2: A methodical study using five types of attachment. Clin Oral Implants Res 2001;12:640–647.
9. Naert I, Quirynen M, Hooghe M, van Steenberghe D. A comparative prospective study of splinted and unsplinted Brånemark implants in mandibular overdenture therapy: A preliminary report. J Prosthet Dent 1994;72:144–151.
10. Jemt T, Harnett J, Heath M, et al. A 5-year prospective multicenter follow-up report on overdentures supported by osseointegrated implants. Int J Oral Maxillofac Implants 1996;11:291–298.
11. Versteegh PA, van Beek GJ, Slagter AP, Ottervanger JP. Clinical evaluation of mandibular overdentures supported by multiple-bar fabrication: A follow-up study of two implant systems. Int J Oral Maxillofac Implants 1995;10:595–603.

12. Naert I, Gizani S, Vuylsteke M, van Steenberghe D. A randomised clinical trial on the influence of splinted and unsplinted oral implants in the mandibular overdenture therapy: A 3-year report. Clin Oral Invest 1997;1:81–88.

13. Gotfredsen K, Holm B. Implant-supported mandibular overdentures retained with ball or bar attachments: A randomized prospective 5-year study. Int J Prosthodont 2000;13:125–130.

14. Naert I, Gizani S, Vuylsteke M, van Steenberghe D. A 5-year randomised clinical trial on the influence of splinted and unsplinted oral implants in the mandibular overdenture therapy. Part I: Peri-implant outcome. Clin Oral Implants Res 1998;9:170–177.

15. Naert I, De Clercq M, Theuniers G, Schepers E. Overdentures supported by osseointegrated fixtures for the edentulous mandible: A 2.5 year report. Int J Oral Maxillofac Implants 1988;3:191–196.

16. Helkimo M. Epidemiological surveys of dysfunction of the masticatory system. In: Zarb GA, Carlsson GE (eds). Temporomandibular Joint Function and Dysfunction. Munksgaard, Copenhagen, 1979:175–192.

17. Naert I, Quirynen M, van Steenberghe D, Duchateau L, Darius P. A comparative study between Brånemark and IMZ implants supporting overdentures: Prosthetic considerations. In: Laney WR, Tolman DE (eds). Tissue Integration in Oral Orthopaedic and Maxillofacial Reconstruction. Chicago: Quintessence, 1990:179–193.

18. Naert I, Hooghe M, Quirynen M, van Steenberghe D. The reliability of implant-retained hinging overdentures for the fully edentulous mandible. An up to 9-year longitudinal study. Clin Oral Invest 1997; 1:119–124.

19. Davis DM, Packer ME. Mandibular overdentures stabilized by Astra Tech implants with either ball attachments or magnets: 5-year results. Int J Prosthodont 1999;12:222–229.

20. Adell R, Lekholm U, Rockler B, et al. Marginal tissue reactions at osseointegrated titanium fixtures. Part I. A 3-year longitudinal prospective study. Int J Oral Maxillofac Surg 1986;1:39–52.

21. Cox JF, Zarb GA. The longitudinal clinical efficacy of osseointegrated dental implants. A 3-year report. Int J Oral Maxillofac Implants 1987;2:91–100.

22. Quirynen M, Naert I, van Steenberghe D, Nys L. A study of 589 consecutive implants supporting complete fixed prostheses. Part I: Periodontal aspects. J Prosthet Dent 1992;68:655–663.

23. Quirynen M, van Steenberghe D, Jacobs R, et al. The reliability of pocket probing around screw-type implants. Clin Oral Implants Res 1991; 2:186–192.

24. Meijer HJA, Kuper JH, Starmans FJM, Bosman F. Stress distribution around dental implants: Influence of superstructure, length of implants, height of mandible. J Prosthet Dent 1992;68:96–101.

25. van Steenberghe D, Quirynen M, Calberson L, Demanet M. Prospective evaluation of the fate of 697 consecutive intra-oral fixtures ad modum Brånemark in the rehabilitation of edentulism. J Head Neck Pathol 1987;6:53–58

26. Engquist B, Bergendall T, Kallus T, Linden U. A retrospective multicenter evaluation of osseointegrated implants supporting overdentures. Int J Oral Maxillofac Implants 1988;3:129–134.

27. Mericske-Stern R. Clinical evaluation of overdenture restorations supported by osseointegrated titanium implants: A retrospective study. Int J Oral Maxillofac Implants 1990;5:375–383.

28. Quirynen M, Naert I, van Steenberghe D, et al. Periodontal aspects of Brånemark and IMZ implants supporting overdentures: A comparative study. In: Laney WR, Tolman DE (eds). Tissue Integration in Oral Orthopaedic and Maxillofacial Reconstruction. Chicago: Quintessence, 1990:80–92.

29. Arvidson K, Bystedt H, Frykholm A, et al. A 3-year clinical study of Astra dental implants in the treatment of edentulous mandibles. Int J Oral Maxillofac Implants 1992;7:321–329.

30. Petropoulos V, Smith W, Kousvelati E. Comparison of retention and release periods for implant overdenture attachments. Int J Oral Maxillofac Implants 1997;12:176–185.

31. Hooghe M, Naert I. Implant-supported overdentures: The Leuven experience. J Dent 1997;25:25–35.

32. van Kampen FMC, van der Bilt A, Cune MS, Bosman F. The influence of various attachment types in mandibular implant-retained overdentures on maximum bite force and EMG. J Dent Res 2002;81: 170–173.

CHAPTER 12

Loading Strategies for Mandibular Implant Overdentures

Alan G. T. Payne, Andrew Tawse-Smith, W. Murray Thomson, and Warwick J. Duncan

The quality of life of elderly edentulous patients can be improved using mandibular interforaminal implants to overcome the edentulous predicament.[1] There is consensus that pairs of splinted or unsplinted implants in the anterior mandible, regardless of the implant system used, are clinically successful, economically advantageous, and structurally sufficient to support an overdenture.[2–5] It has also become acceptable to place implants in one stage using the nonsubmerged approach,[6,7] or by modification of the original two-stage submerged procedure.[8–10] As a result, implant placement protocols now require fewer costly surgical procedures.

At one time, it was recommended that a 12-week healing period be allowed prior to loading of implants. Now it is generally accepted that premature functional loading[11] of splinted or unsplinted mandibular implants with overdentures can occur before completion of the conventional 12-week healing period. There are three approaches to premature loading. Early loading describes placement of a prosthesis before 12 weeks, usually after 1 week, but within a period of 20 to 28 days after im-

plant placement.[8] Progressive loading describes the gradual increase in force on a dental implant whether applied intentionally with a prosthesis or unintentionally via forces placed by adjacent anatomic structures or parafunctional loading.[12] With immediate loading, full occlusal and incisal loading is placed on a dental implant with the prosthesis the same day as surgery or within the first few days after surgery.[12]

Critical determinants of any premature functional loading strategy are related to primary implant stability and an absence of micromotion at surgery, bone type, implant length, and implant surface.[11] Implant success with these approaches is achieved with a functional prosthesis in an absence of discomfort, altered sensation, or infection; evidence of minimal marginal bone loss; and implant stability.[13]

Early loading of implants with either the original smooth (turned) surfaces or, more recently, different roughened surfaces is a paradigm shift welcomed by clinicians.[14,15] With early loading, the original 12-week healing period prior to loading can be systematically shortened[11] to expedite an earlier improvement in masticatory function and quality of life for elderly edentulous patients.[16]

The evaluation of different early loading protocols for unsplinted implants for mandibular overdentures opposing conventional complete maxillary dentures is best achieved by comparing groups with different reductions in healing times. The Clinical Overdenture Research Project, School of Dentistry, University of Otago, Dunedin, New Zealand, has conducted a controlled prospective clinical trial on edentulous patients using four different implant types (ITI Dental Implant System, Straumann, Waldenburg, Switzerland; Brånemark System or Steri-Oss, Nobel Biocare, Göteborg, Sweden; and Southern Implants, Irene, South Africa) to determine the minimum safe interval between placement and functional loading of unsplinted implants supporting mandibular overdentures that oppose conventional maxillary complete dentures. This study demonstrated that early functional loading of implants with mandibular overdentures at 2 or 6 weeks after implant placement is an effective treatment for edentulous patients.

Clinical Overdenture Study

Patient Selection

One hundred and six edentulous patients (mean age 65.3 years, SD 7.4) with a history of difficulties with their complete dentures and between 8 and 15 mm of residual anterior mandibular bone were selected using standard inclusion and exclusion criteria.[17] Overall, 38% of the patients were men, although there were higher numbers of men in the Southern 6-week group (58.3%), ITI 6-week group (66.7%), and ITI 2-week group (50%). Patients had been edentulous for a mean period of 34.7 years (SD 13.4), and most had worn more than three sets of replacement complete

dentures. Groups did not differ significantly by age, number of years of edentulousness, or number of previous dentures. On average, each set of complete dentures had been worn for 11.2 years (SD 6.8), and implant length ranged from 8.5 to 18 mm. The majority of patients had either type II or III bone quantity, with type C or D bone quality. The groups were similar in implant length, bone quality, and quantity.

Using a table of random numbers, patients were randomly allocated[18] to be treated using one of four different implant systems. One of these systems used implants with a machined smooth titanium implant surface (Brånemark). The other three systems offered implants with roughened titanium surfaces to varying extents (Steri-Oss, ITI, and Southern Implants). An attempt was made for each implant system to have a control group (12 weeks healing) and two test groups (6 and 2 weeks healing). Twelve patients were allocated to each group, except for the 2-week Brånemark group, to which only 10 patients were assigned. Treatment planning included preoperative diagnostic panoramic radiographs (Scanora, Soridex, Orion, Helsinki, Finland), conventional lateral cephalometric radiographs, and new maxillary and mandibular complete dentures.

Surgical and Prosthodontic Procedures

Treatment regimes (Figs 12-1 and 12-2) allowed the following implants to be placed with the same equipment using a standardized one-stage approach: two Steri-Oss HL Series acid-etched machined titanium implants (diameter 3.8 mm); two Southern sandblasted acid-etched titanium implants (diameter 3.75 mm); or two conical smooth (turned) titanium Brånemark implants (diameter 3.75 mm).[8–10] The ITI sandblasted, large-grit, acid-etched (SLA) implants

12-week healing group	6-week healing group	2-week healing group
Steri-Oss, 3.8-mm machined ITI, 4.1-mm SLA surface Southern, 3.75-mm surface-enhanced	Steri-Oss, 3.8-mm machined ITI, 4.1-mm SLA surface Southern, 3.75-mm surface-enhanced	Brånemark, 3.75-mm machined ITI, 4.1-mm SLA surface Southern, 3.75-mm surface-enhanced

Two mandibular implants placed
(One-stage surgical protocol)

Healing abutment Steri-Oss, 7 mm ITI, 3 mm Southern, 6 mm	*Healing abutment* Steri-Oss, 7 mm ITI, 3 mm Southern, 6 mm	*Permanent abutment* Brånemark, ball ITI, retentive anchor Southern, ball
Healing period 12 weeks	Healing period 6 weeks	Healing period 2 weeks
Permanent abutment Steri-Oss, ball ITI, retentive anchor Southern, ball	*Permanent abutment* Steri-Oss, ball ITI, retentive anchor Southern, ball	

Fit matrices in denture
Closed-mouth reline impression
Stability tests and standardized radiographs at 6 or 12 weeks
Peri-implant parameters recorded at specific time points

Repeat clinical measurements annually for up to 3 years
Prosthodontic maintenance

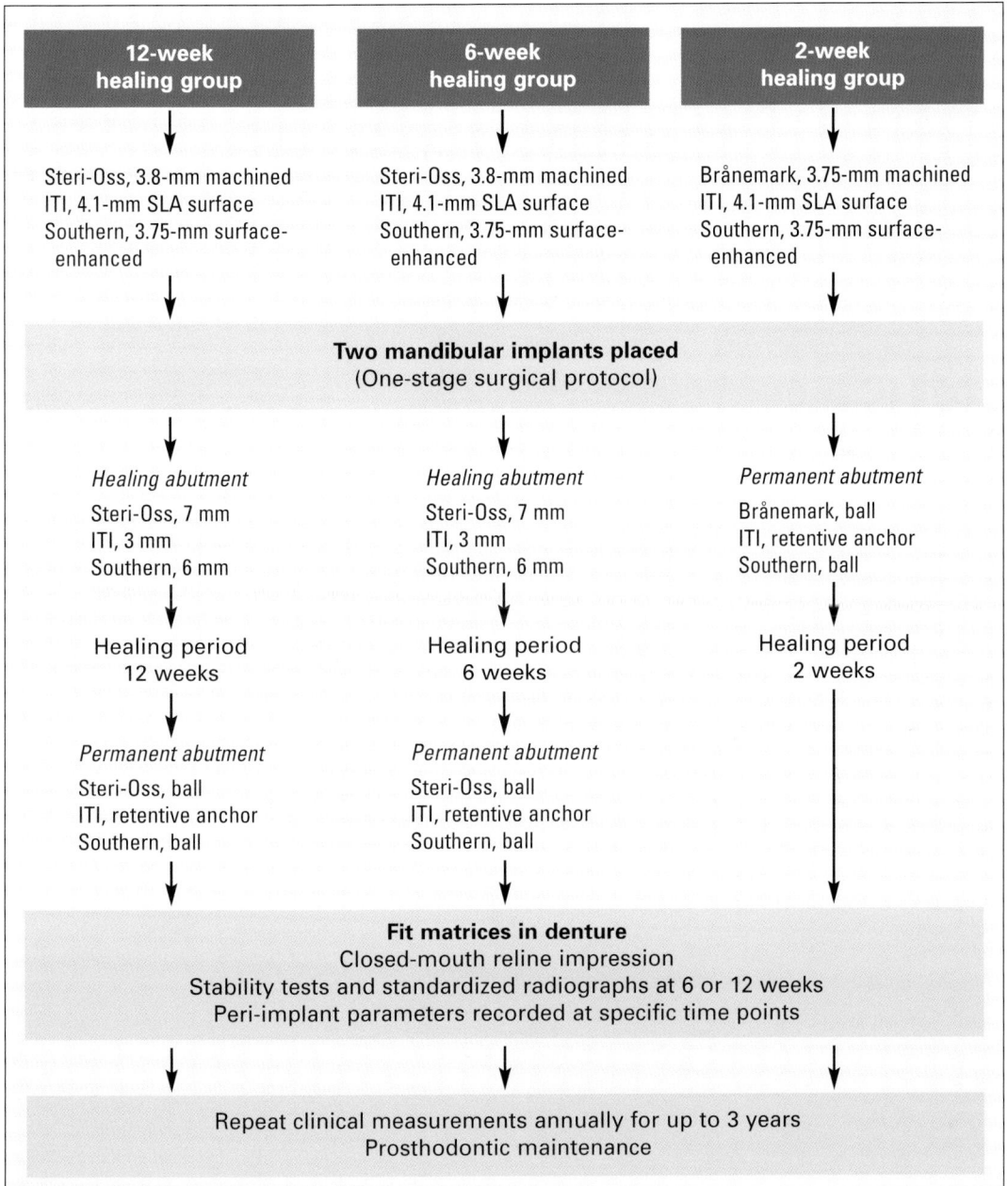

Fig 12-1 Treatment protocols for the three loading groups.

Fig 12-2 Panoramic radiographs of the four implant systems placed in patients. (Figures 12-2a and 12-2b are reprinted with permission from Tawse-Smith et al.[19] Figure 12-2d is reprinted with permission from Payne et al.[20])

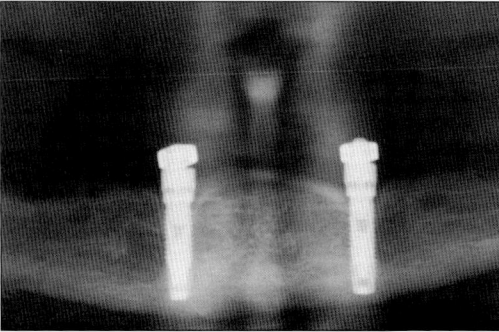

Fig 12-2a Steri-Oss HL series implants, 3.8-mm diameter with O-ring abutments.

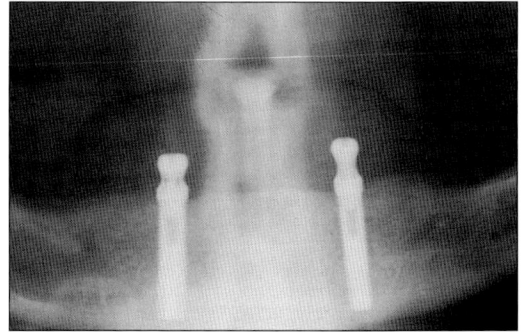

Fig 12-2b Southern implants, 3.75-mm diameter with standard ball abutments.

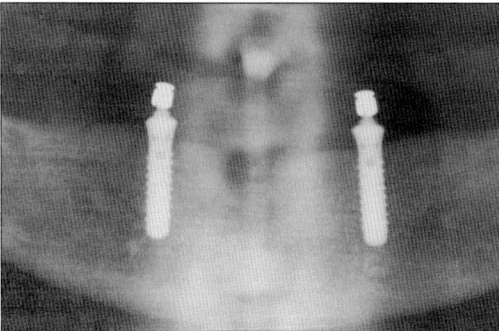

Fig 12-2c ITI implants, 4.1-mm diameter with retentive anchors.

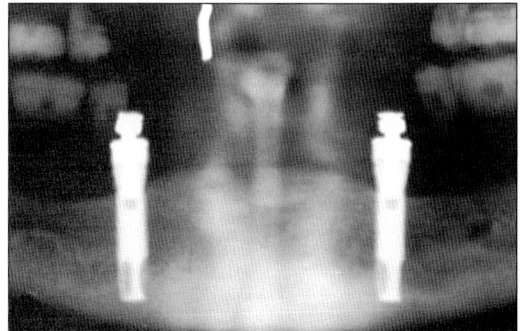

Fig 12-2d Brånemark conical implants, 3.75-mm diameter with mini 2.25-mm ball abutments.

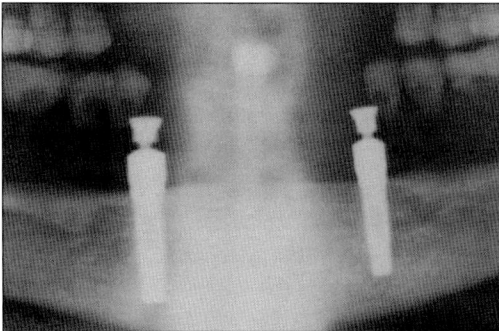

Fig 12-2e Southern implants, 3.75-mm diameter with mini 2.25-mm ball abutments.

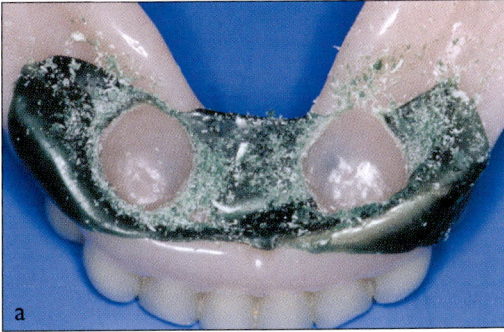

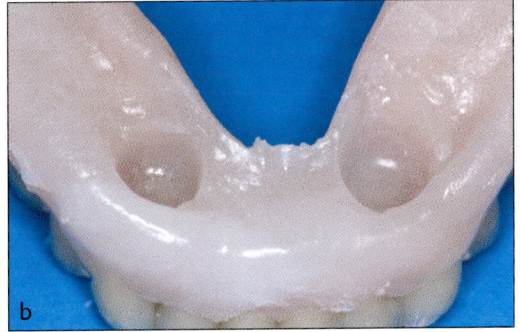

Figs 12-3a and 12-3b Tissue conditioning for the 12-week and 6-week groups at 10 to 14 days. *(a)* Denture preparation. *(b)* Tissue conditioner in existing denture.

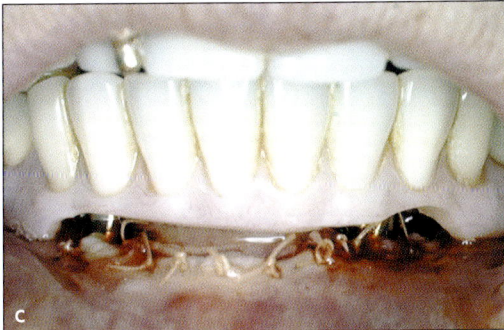

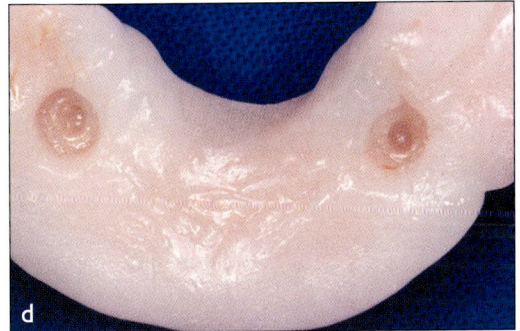

Figs 12-3c and 12-3d Tissue conditioning for the 2-week group at the time of surgery. *(c)* Denture relief. *(d)* Tissue conditioner in existing denture. (Figure 12-3c is reprinted with permission from Payne et al.[20])

(diameter 4.1 mm) were placed with a non-submerged one-stage protocol.[7] Bicortical anchorage and primary stability was mandatory.

Patients in the 12-week and 6-week groups did not wear their mandibular denture for 10 days, after which time tissue conditioner was applied to its undersurface to minimize loading forces (Figs 12-3a and 12-3b). Patients in the 2-week healing groups were permitted to use their mandibular dentures immediately postoperatively (Figs 12-3c and 12-3d), with a soft diet for the first 2 weeks, and they were given strict instructions to remove the prosthesis at night. The postoperative care protocol included daily 0.2% chlorhexidine rinses and peri-implant application of chlorhexidine gel (Perioguard, Colgate Oral Care, Sydney, Australia), using the

denture as a reservoir. After specific healing periods, each mandibular denture was relined to include respective matrices (Fig 12-4).

Follow-up Procedures

Implant stability tests using either the Periotest device (Siemens AG, Bensheim, Germany) or the Osstell device (Integration Diagnostics, Göteborg, Sweden) were performed at baseline and specified annual intervals postinsertion. Standardized intraoral radiographs of the coronal parts of the implants were taken with a modified technique[22] and marginal bone changes were measured by two calibrated examiners using 7x magnification (Fig 12-5). For all 6- and 12-week healing groups, the peri-

Fig 12-4 Prosthodontic retentive components of the four implant systems. (Figures 12-4a to 12-4c are reprinted with permission from Watson et al.[21] Figure 12-4d is reprinted with permission from Payne et al.[20])

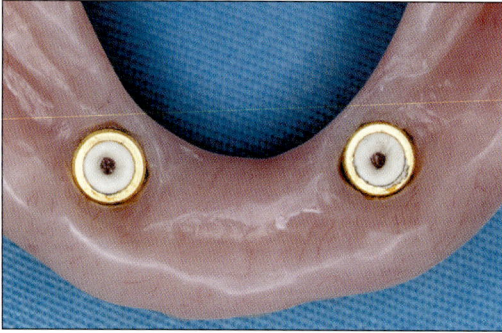

Fig 12-4a Steri-Oss rubber O-ring matrices.

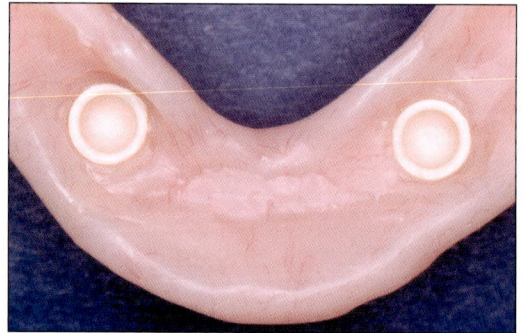

Fig 12-4b Southern plastic cap matrices.

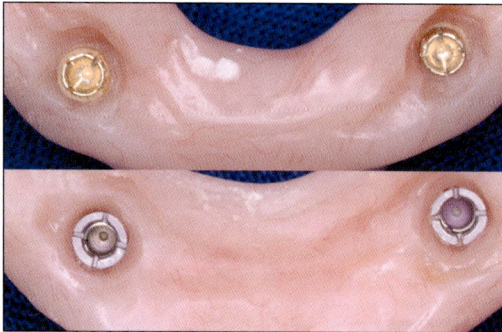

Fig 12-4c ITI gold matrices and titanium matrices with stainless steel spring.

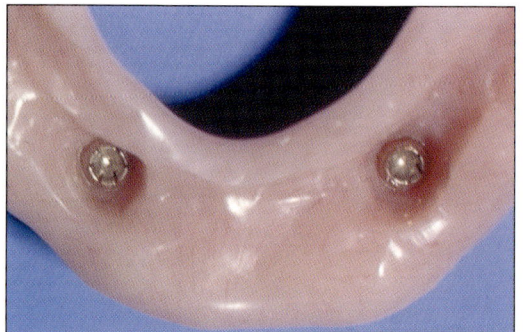

Fig 12-4d Brånemark gold alloy matrices.

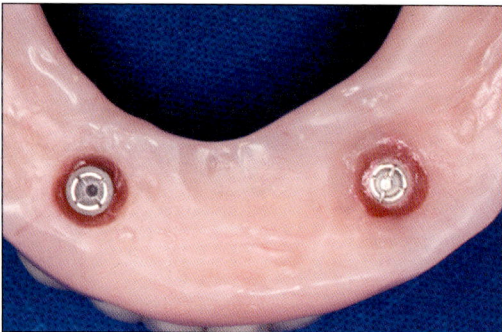

Fig 12-4e Southern palladium matrices.

Fig 12-5 Standardized radiographs. (Figure 12-5b is reprinted with permission from Payne et al.[23] Figure 12-5e is reprinted with permission from Payne et al.[20])

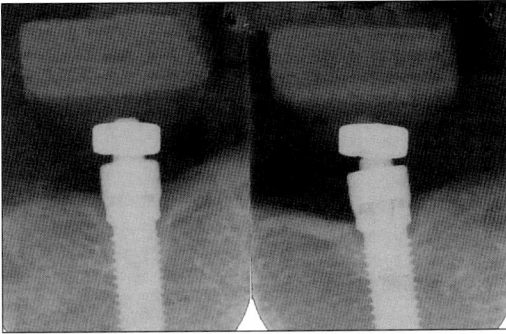

Fig 12-5a Steri-Oss implant and O-ring abutment.

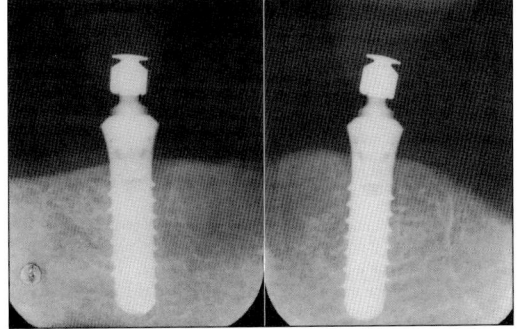

Fig 12-5b ITI implant and retentive anchor.

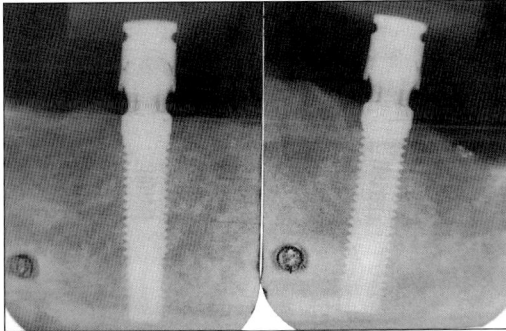

Fig 12-5c Southern implant and standard abutment.

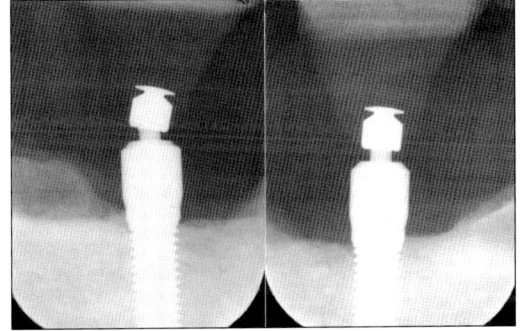

Fig 12-5d Southern implant and mini 2.25-mm ball abutment.

Fig 12-5e Brånemark implant and mini 2.25-mm ball abutment.

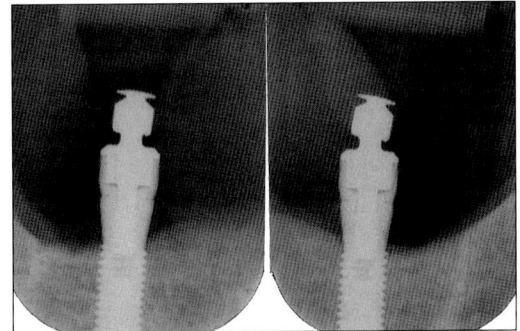

implant parameters using periodontal techniques were measured 4 weeks after patrix placement, at 10 and 16 weeks, respectively. For all 2-week healing groups, the peri-implant parameters were taken at 6 weeks to first allow for mucosal maturation. The shoulder of each implant (ITI and Brånemark), the top of the abutment cylinder (Steri-Oss), or the top of the ball abutment (Southern) were used as the reference points. Standardized oral hygiene instructions with end-tufted toothbrushes or powered brushes[24] were provided after abutment connection and were reinforced at recall appointments; professional cleaning also was performed at recall appointments. Patients were followed for up to 3 years after implant placement for evaluation of implant success rates.[13]

Data Analysis

At each patient recall, changes in marginal bone levels on radiographs were computed both mesially and distally from the reference point, enabling calculation of the marginal bone loss over time. Success rates by implant type and loading strategy at the patient level were computed by determining whether it met the stage-specific criteria for success.[25] Mean values were computed for implant stability measurements and for peri-implant parameters for each examination and were compared using the Wilcoxon test for related samples. Differences in proportions were tested for statistical significance using the chi-square test (or the McNemar test when change over time was examined). Differences between the implant types were tested for significance using the independent samples t test.

Success of Early Loading

Patient Exclusions and Implant Failure

The 6-week and 2-week healing groups did not show any significant differences from the 12-week groups in success rate. In the Steri-Oss 12-week group, only one patient had an early failure (one implant). In the Steri-Oss 6-week group, six patients had a total of seven early implant failures. During the follow-up evaluations, lower success rate levels were seen for both the 12-week and 6-week Steri-Oss groups compared to their Southern Implant counterparts. One patient in the Steri-Oss 12-week group requested to be excluded from the study after the 2-year recall, and two patients from the Southern 12-week group emigrated and missed the 2-year recall, but returned for the 3-year recall. The failed Steri-Oss implants all had been placed by the same surgeon. At the 2- and 3-year recalls, only one set of radiographs for one patient in the Southern 6-week group was unreadable. Two patients in the ITI 12-week group were not available for follow-up at years 1, 2, and 3 because of emigration. Almost all the 34 patients in the 2-week groups were recalled at the 1-year appointment, except one patient of the ITI group, who was unable to attend due to medical reasons. There were no late implant failures up to the 3-year recall visits for any of the treatment groups. Marginal bone loss over the study was in the range of 0.1 to 0.4 mm during the first year, and these numbers decreased in subsequent years with some evidence of marginal bone gain.

Implant Stability Tests

The Periotest instrument showed increasingly negative values, which indicated stability of all implants for all 12-week and 6-week groups. The Osstell resonance frequency analyses were taken at the end of year 2 for the Southern and ITI 12-week and 6-week groups; there were no statistically significant differences between these two groups. Apart from the Brånemark 2-week group, all implant stability tests for the 2-week patients (Southern and ITI) were taken with resonance frequency analysis. There was a significant difference in the resonance frequency values during follow-up between the Southern and ITI 2-week healing groups, with higher values in the Southern group (range of implant stability quotient: 58.4 to 73.4).

Peri-implant Responses

For the Steri-Oss and Southern 6-week and 12-week healing groups, there was an excellent peri-implant mucosal response following the one-stage surgical approach with healing abutments (Figs 12-6a and 12-6b), after patrix placement at baseline and at 1 year (Figs 12-6c to 12-6f). For all ITI, Southern, and Brånemark 2-week healing groups with placement of the patrices at surgery, the peri-implant response also progressed favorably up to 1 year (Figs 12-7 to 12-9).

Postoperative mucosal swelling was evident for the 12-week and 6-week groups for all implant systems tested, but this swelling subsided during the respective healing periods. In the 2-week groups, postoperative mucosal swelling was seen in 17% of the Southern group (2 of 12 patients), 50% of the ITI group (6 of 12 patients) and 40% of the Brånemark 2-week patients (4 of 10 patients). This swelling subsided after the 2-week healing period and did not interfere with early prosthodontic reline procedures. Analysis of soft tissue parameters by implant systems over time revealed no statistically significant differences at baseline, 1, 2, or 3 years postplacement. The polished coronal necks of some ITI implants were positioned below the alveolar crest; as a result, probing depths increased slightly with time around this implant system and some minimal mucosal problems (mucosal enlargement or overgrowth) were seen. Perimucosal inflammation and plaque scores remained low throughout the observation period for all implant systems. Narrow zones of keratinized mucosa (less than 2 mm) were common among all groups through the end of the study period.

Fig 12-6 Examples of changes in peri-implant soft tissues, following one-stage surgery, throughout the observation period for the 12-week and 6-week groups. (Figures 12-6a to 12-6d are reprinted with permission from Tawse-Smith.[10] Figures 12-6e and 12-6f are reprinted with permission from Tawse-Smith.[19])

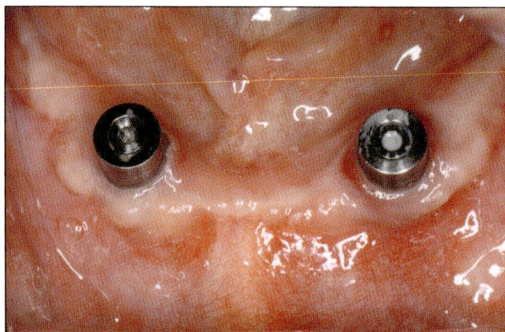

Fig 12-6a Southern implants (healing abutments) at 12 weeks.

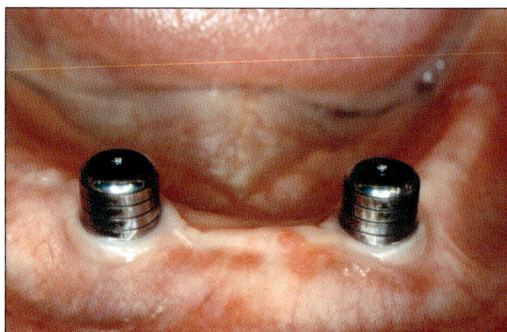

Fig 12-6b Steri-Oss implants (healing abutments) at 12 weeks.

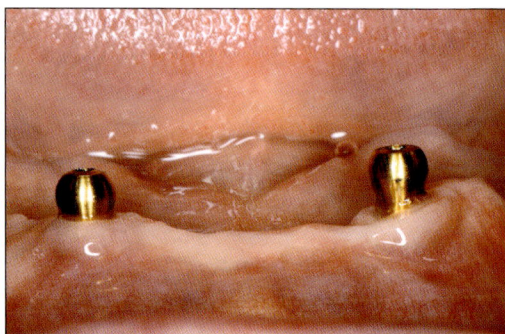

Fig 12-6c Southern implants (standard ball abutment) at baseline.

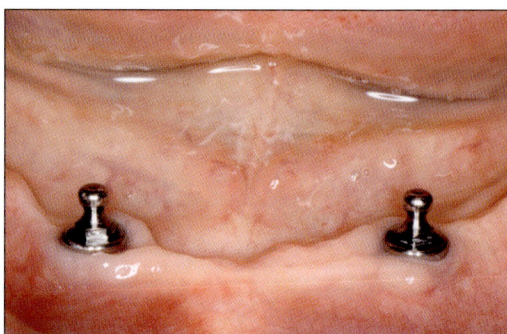

Fig 12-6d Steri-Oss implants at baseline.

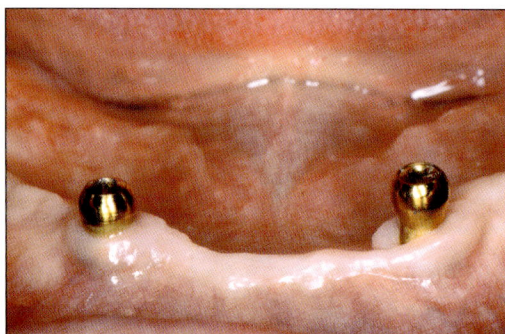

Fig 12-6e Southern implants (standard ball abutment) at 1 year.

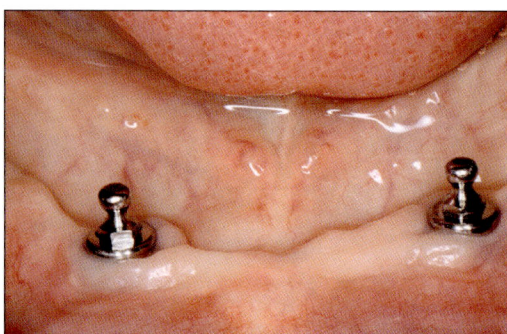

Fig 12-6f Steri-Oss implants at 1 year.

Fig 12-7 Examples of changes in peri-implant soft tissues throughout the observation period for the 2-week ITI groups.

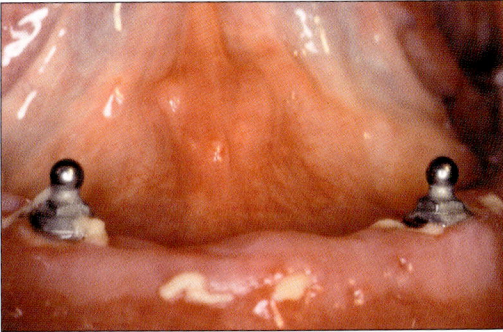

Fig 12-7a One week postoperatively.

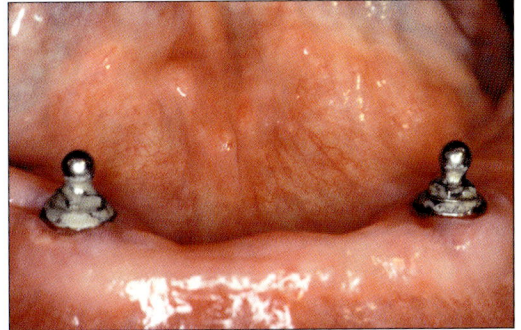

Fig 12-7b Two weeks postoperatively.

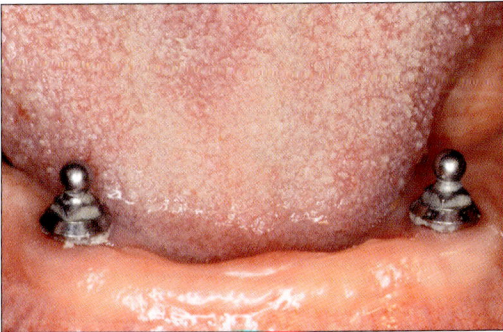

Fig 12-7c Six weeks postoperatively.

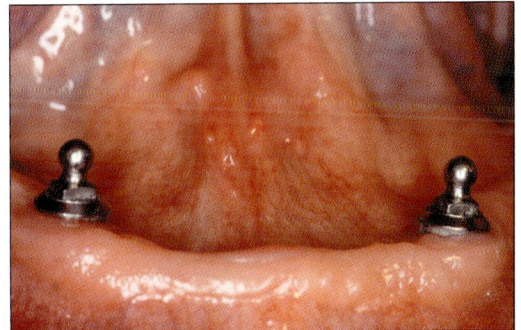

Fig 12-7d One year postoperatively.

Fig 12-8 Examples of changes in peri-implant soft tissues throughout the observation period for 2-week Southern implant (with mini 2.25-mm ball abutments) groups.

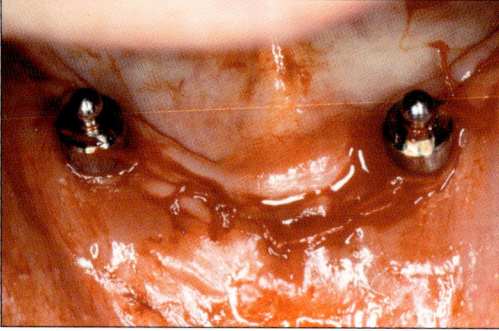

Fig 12-8a Immediately postoperatively.

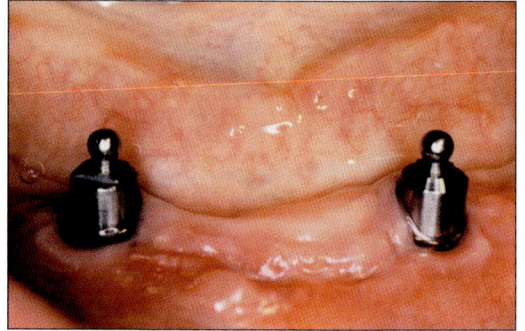

Fig 12-8b Two weeks postoperatively.

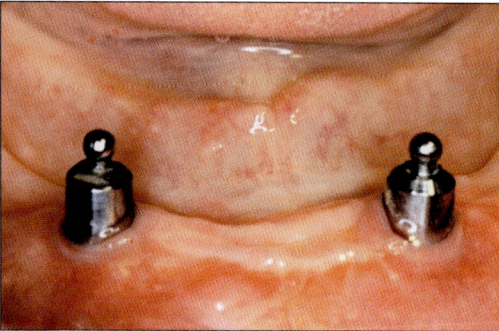

Fig 12-8c Twelve weeks postoperatively.

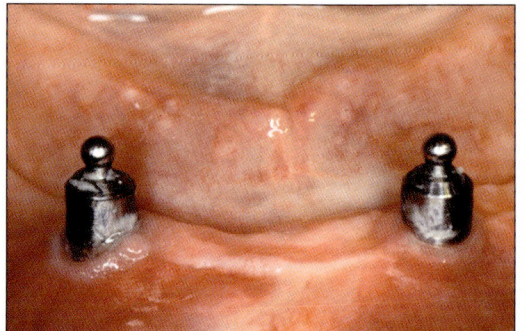

Fig 12-8d One year postoperatively.

Fig 12-9 Examples of changes in peri-implant soft tissues throughout the observation period for 2-week Bränemark (with mini 2.25-mm ball abutment) group. (Reprinted with permission from Payne et al.[20])

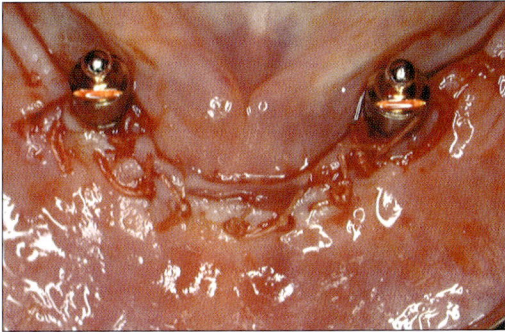

Fig 12-9a Immediately postoperatively.

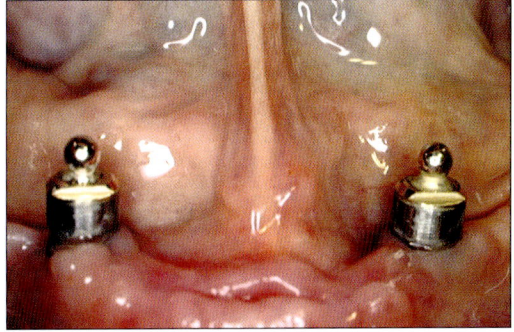

Fig 12-9b Two weeks postoperatively.

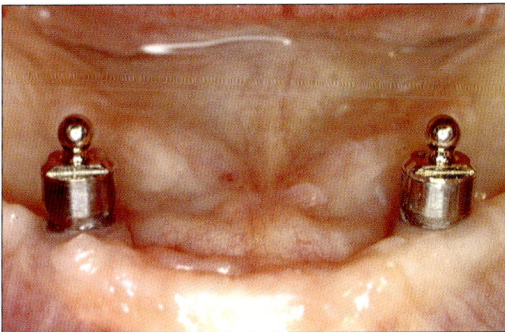

Fig 12-9c Twelve weeks postoperatively.

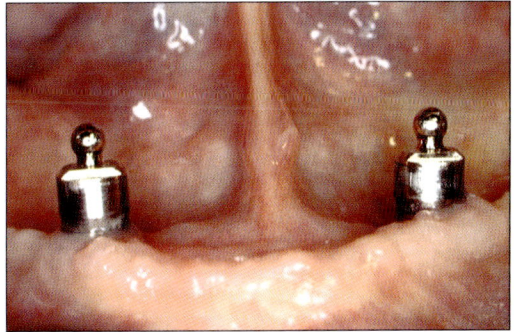

Fig 12-9d One year postoperatively.

Table 12-1 Prosthodontic maintenance events during the first year after loading (n denotes number of patients)

Categories	All maintenance events* (n = 106)	No. of maintenance events per implant group						
		12- and 6-week groups combined				2-week groups		
		Steri-Oss, Rubber O-ring (n = 24)	Southern, plastic matrix (n = 24)	ITI titanium matrix (n = 12)	ITI gold matrix (n = 12)	Southern palladium matrix (n = 12)	ITI gold matrix (n = 12)	Brånemark gold matrix (n = 10)
Patrix screw fracture	1					1		
Patrix loose	6	3				3		
Matrix or its respective housing dislodged or worn	33	18		7	3	4		1
Matrix activated	71				18	18	19	16
Matrix replaced	102	58	20	23	1			
Matrix fractured	11			9	1			1
Fractured implant overdenture, puncture fracture of acrylic over patrix, or fracture of denture teeth	8		3		3	1	1	
Reline overdenture	22		6	4	6	2	2	2
New overdenture	1			1				
Maxillary denture—retention complaints	7		6		1			
Maxillary denture—reline	7		5			1	1	
Maxillary denture adjustment—phonetic complaints	5	2	3					
Maxillary denture adjustment—esthetic complaints	2	1	1					
Lip/cheek biting complaints	3	2	1					
Total	**279**	84	45	44	33	30	23	21

*For both mandibular overdenture and maxillary denture.

Prosthodontic Maintenance Requirements

All 106 patients were able to wear their existing dentures and to masticate comfortably, with the tissue conditioner in place during the 2-, 6- or 12-week healing periods. In the 2-week healing groups, patient-identified discomfort warranted adjustment of the contour of the tissue conditioner on the overdenture in only 20% of patients. There were no statistically significant differences in prosthodontic maintenance events (regardless of matrix design) during the first year with different loading strategies (Table 12-1). The number of relines required during the first year was not significantly greater for the 2-week healing groups (24%) than for the other 6- or 12-week groups (22%).

Long-term Clinical Implications of Early Loading

The outcome of this clinical trial indicates that there are no adverse consequences for either smooth machined (turned) titanium or roughened-surface titanium implants being loaded with mandibular overdentures as early as 2 weeks. The findings of this study also suggest that early-loaded implants placed in the anterior mandible and used as support for overdentures can succeed in both type II and type III bone. There may be no need to limit this treatment approach to type I bone only, as has been previously recommended.[11] It appears that, in view of the wide range of implant systems used, careful, controlled surgical placement is more important than implant length. The critical determinant of implant success in the anterior mandible is undoubtedly primary implant stability and the absence of micromotion, in contrast to the osseous quality or biomaterial microsurface reported in other stud-

ies.[11,19,26] Excessive interfacial micromotion postimplantation interferes with local bone healing, may cause a fibrous tissue interface, and may prevent the fibrin clot from adhering to the implant surface during early healing.[11]

Monitoring Marginal Bone Loss

The use of standardized radiographs at each scheduled follow-up has allowed measurement and monitoring of marginal bone changes surrounding early-loaded unsplinted implants, although direct comparison between systems at each assessment is difficult because of the use of different reference points. However, assessing and comparing changes in bone level over time eliminated this problem, and illustrated that there were no significant differences in this parameter among implant systems or loading strategies. Marginal bone loss in this study compared well with other mandibular overdenture studies using conventional 12-week loading periods.[3,4,6] It is recommended that a periapical radiograph be taken of each implant at each recall appointment to help the clinician monitor changes in bone level.

Variability of Testing Mechanisms

The improvement of implant stability readings through the study period indicated continuous bone contact with the implant surfaces. This study's Periotest values at 6 weeks for early-loaded Steri-Oss, Southern, and SLA-surface implants are within accepted values. The authors had great difficulty detecting differences between mobile and rigid implants using the Periotest because of the device's narrow working range. After 1 year, the method of measurement was changed to resonance frequency analysis (RFA) for measurement of implant stability. However, to date, only the diagnostic, and not prognostic, value has been demonstrated for this technique. The RFA values of this study are similar to those reported for other implant systems used in the anterior mandible, albeit those RFA values were for fixed implant prostheses.[9]

Ramifications of Peri-implant Mucosal Health

The peri-implant parameters highlighted in this chapter are similar to those from other reports on implant-supported overdentures.[5] These data also suggest that, regardless of implant design, a minimum of 2 mm of keratinized mucosa is not essential for maintenance of soft tissue health. Learning experiences with the ITI implants resulted in more mucosal problems than should be necessary and led researchers to identify the differences in surgical protocols between the systems. The need for systematic collection of data on peri-implant soft tissue parameters during overdenture clinical trials has been questioned.[4] However, a review of the relevant literature revealed that 60% of studies of mandibular overdentures supported by implants reported gingival hyperplasia or mucosal enlargement underneath the prosthesis.[27] The authors feel that there is insufficient evidence, at this stage, to ignore the possibility that a pathogenic flora may increase the risk of implant failure when provided with an appropriate environmental niche underneath overdentures supported by implants in a susceptible host. Because of this, they have chosen to monitor peri-implant mucosal health. The findings reveal that well-motivated patients and a sound recall program can result in low levels of perimucosal inflammation, which increases the chances of long-term peri-implant health for aging edentulous patients who have been rehabilitated with overdentures. The low mean bleeding index scores and the improvement in mean plaque scores over

the study period reflect patient cooperation. However, only a small number of patients were able to maintain sites that were entirely free of plaque accumulation, which indicates the oral hygiene challenge for patients. This is despite an intensive postoperative oral hygiene program as a result of an investigation into the oral self-care of these same patients.[24]

Use of Tissue Conditioners with Immediate Loading

Although tissue conditioner and generous relief of the overdenture were provided around the healing abutments in the 12- and 6-week groups (where a one-stage surgical approach was used), there was still a possibility of early overloading. The authors acknowledge that some progressive loading[12] in the 2-week healing groups would have also occurred when the tissue conditioner directly contacted the superior and lateral surfaces of the ball abutments when overdenture wear occurred immediately following surgical placement.[20] None of the patients found it necessary to remove their modified mandibular denture because of postoperative discomfort, which perhaps is due to use of tissue-conditioning material. The application of tissue conditioner postsurgically for the 2-week group was clinically demanding because of the presence of clotting blood and sutures. When the implant systems included different abutments with a range of heights, longer abutments were deliberately selected at surgery to limit the infringement of postoperative mucosal swelling. Choosing a ball abutment that was high enough to avoid postoperative soft tissue overgrowth, and yet low enough to avoid forces during initial function with progressive loading, is a problem when a clinician uses this treatment approach. Since support for mandibular overdentures supported by two implants is provided by both the mucosa and the implants, immediate loading[12] with the matrices inserted in the denture on the day of surgery may be precluded. A mandatory 2-week mucosal healing period prior to including the matrices in the overdenture is proposed.

Conclusions

A nonsubmerged surgical procedure for ITI and conical Brånemark implants, or a one-stage surgical procedure for Steri-Oss and Southern implants, followed by conventional loading with mandibular overdentures at 12 weeks or early loading at 6 weeks or even 2 weeks, is an effective treatment for edentulous patients. Early loading of mandibular overdentures supported by implants may commence as early as 2 weeks after implant placement for ITI, Brånemark, and Southern implant systems. Mucosal healing prevents loading earlier than 2 weeks postinsertion. Patients undergoing implant overdenture therapy are able to wear their existing mandibular denture with a tissue conditioning material on the undersurface, beginning the day of surgery and continuing during the 2-week postsurgical period. Loading forces are minimized by requesting that patients eat only soft meals for the first 6 weeks.

Acknowledgments

The authors would like to thank the patients and the following staff of the Clinical Overdenture Research Project, School of Dentistry, University of Otago, Dunedin, New Zealand: Dr Rohana Kumara especially is thanked for placing many of the implants, and Drs Gilbert Watson and Dusan Kuzmanovic are acknowledged for the use of their research data.

In addition, Institut Straumann AG and the ITI Foundation Research Grant 2003/RCL 2000, Waldenburg, Switzerland; Nobel Biocare Pty (Ltd), Sydney, Australia; Southern Implants, Irene, South Africa; Ivoclar Vivadent, Auckland, New Zealand; Shalfoon Dental, Dunedin, New Zealand; Colgate Oral Care, Auckland, New Zealand; and Radiographic Supplies Ltd, Christchurch, New Zealand, are acknowledged for their generous support of the study.

References

1. Zarb GA. The edentulous milieu. J Prosthet Dent 1983;49:825–831.
2. Jemt T, Chai J, Harnett J, et al. A 5-year prospective multicenter follow-up report on overdentures supported by osseointegrated implants. Int J Oral Maxillofac Implants 1996;11:291–298.
3. Naert I, Gizani S, Vuylskeke M, van Steenberghe D. A 5-year prospective randomized clinical trial on the influence of splinted and unsplinted oral implants retaining a mandibular overdenture: Prosthetic aspects and patient satisfaction. J Oral Rehabil 1999; 26:195–202.
4. Schmitt A, Zarb GA. The notion of implant-supported overdentures. J Prosthet Dent 1998;79:60–65.
5. Wismeijer D, van Waas MAJ, Mulder J, Vermeeren JJJF, Kalk W. Clinical and radiological results of patients treated with three treatment modalities for overdentures on implants of the ITI Dental Implant System. Clin Oral Implants Res 1999;10:297–306.
6. Mericske-Stern R. Treatment outcomes with implant-supported overdentures: Clinical considerations. J Prosthet Dent 1998;79:66–73.
7. Cochran DL. The scientific basis for and clinical experiences with Staumann implants including the ITI Dental Implant System: A consensus report. Clin Oral Implants Res 2001;11(Suppl 1):33–58.
8. Ericsson I, Randow K, Nilner K, Peterson A. Early functional loading of Brånemark implants. 5-year clinical follow-up study. Clin Implant Dent Relat Res 2000;2:70–77.
9. Friberg B, Sennerby L, Linden B, Grondahl UK, Lekholm U. Stability measurements of one-stage Brånemark implants during healing in mandibles. A clinical resonance frequency analysis study. Int J Oral Maxillofac Surg 1999;28:266–272.
10. Tawse-Smith A, Payne AGT, Kumara R, Thomson WM. A one-stage operative procedure using 2 different implant systems: A prospective study on implant overdentures in the edentulous mandible. Clin Implant Dent Relat Res 2001;3:185–193.

11. Szmukler-Moncler S, Piattelli A, Favero GA, Dubruille JH. Considerations preliminary to the application of early and immediate loading protocols in dental implantology. Clin Oral Implants Res 2000;11:12–25.

12. The Academy of Prosthodontics. The Glossary of Prosthodontic Terms (ed 7). J Prosthet Dent 1999; 81:41–110.

13. Albrektsson T, Zarb GA. Determinants of correct clinical reporting. Int J Prosthodont 1998;11:517–521.

14. Cochran DL. A comparison of endosseous dental implant surfaces. J Periodontol 1999;70:1523–1539.

15. Sul YT, Johansson CB, Jeong Y, Wennerberg A, Albrektsson T. Resonance frequency and removal torque analysis of implants with turned and anodized surface oxides. Clin Oral Implants Res 2002; 13:252–259.

16. Carr AB. Successful long-term treatment outcomes in the field of osseointegrated implants: Prosthodontic determinants. Int J Prosthodont 1998;11: 502–512.

17. Lekholm U, Zarb, GA. Patient selection and preparation. In: Brånemark PI, Zarb GA, Albrektsson T (eds). Tissue Integrated Prostheses: Osseointegration in Clinical Dentistry. Chicago: Quintessence, 1985:199–210.

18. Espositio M, Coulthard P, Worthington HV, Jokstad A. Quality assessment of randomized controlled trials of oral implants. Int J Oral Maxillofac Implants 2000;16:783–792.

19. Tawse-Smith A, Payne AGT, Kumara, R, Thomson WM. Early loading on unsplinted implants supporting mandibular overdentures using a one-stage operative procedure with two different implant systems: A 2-year report. Clin Implant Dent Relat Res 2002;4:33–42.

20. Payne AGT, Tawse-Smith A, Kumara R, Thomson WM. One-year prospective evaluation of the early loading of unsplinted conical Brånemark fixtures with mandibular overdentures: A preliminary report. Clin Implant Dent Relat Res 2001;3:9–18.

21. Watson G, Payne AGT, Purton DG, Thomson WG. Mandibular implant overdentures: Comparative evaluation of the prosthodontic maintenance during the first year of service using three different systems. Int J Prosthodont 2002;15:259–266.

22. Payne AGT, Solomons YF, Lownie JF. Standardization of radiographs for mandibular implant-supported overdentures: Review and innovation. Clin Oral Implants Res 1999;10:307–319.

23. Payne AGT, Tawse-Smith A, Duncan W, Kumara R. Early loading of unsplinted ITI implants supporting mandibular overdentures: Two-year results of a randomized controlled trial. Clin Oral Implants Res 2002;13:603–609.

24. Tawse-Smith A, Duncan W, Payne AGT, Thomson WM, Wennström JL. Effectiveness of electric toothbrushes in peri-implant maintenance of mandibular implant overdentures. J Clin Periodontol 2002;29: 275–280.

25. Fourmousis I, Bragger U. Radiographic interpretation of peri-implant structures. In: Lang NP, Karring T, Lindhe J (eds). Proceedings of the 3rd European Workshop on Periodontology–Implant Dentistry. Chicago: Quintessence, 1999:228–241.

26. Payne AGT, Tawse-Smith A, Duncan WJ, Kumara R. Conventional and early loading of unsplinted ITI implants supporting mandibular overdentures: Two-year results of a prospective randomized clinical trial. Clin Oral Implants Res 2002;13:603–609.

27. Payne AGT, Solomons YF, Lownie JF, Tawse-Smith A. Inter-abutment and peri-abutment mucosal enlargement with mandibular implant overdentures. Clin Oral Implants Res 2001;13:179–187.

CHAPTER 13

Two-Implant Overdentures with Ball Attachments: A Step-by-Step Approach

Pierre Boudrias and Antoine Chehade

Dental implants are widely used as anchors for various types of implant-supported prostheses. Mandibular overdentures supported by two implants provide greater patient satisfaction, chewing ability, and comfort compared to conventional dentures.[1-4] An anterior short bar or single attachments (ball attachments, magnets, and O-rings) have been used successfully to improve overdenture retention.[5-7] This chapter illustrates the step-by-step surgical and prosthetic procedures in the fabrication of a ball-retained mandibular overdenture supported by two implants.

Treatment Considerations

Overdenture therapy is indicated[1] for:

1. Patients who are dissatisfied with complete dentures and demand greater stability and oral comfort.
2. Elderly patients who desire a more stable mandibular denture.

3. Patients who have congenital or oral and maxillofacial defects and are in need of oral rehabilitation.

For patients with difficulty functioning and adapting to a mandibular conventional denture, two standard-diameter implants at least 10 mm in length are generally sufficient to provide retention and support for an overdenture prosthesis.[8,9]

Patients who wear conventional dentures for a long period have a greater chance of developing problems, especially with the mandibular prosthesis, due to unfavorable loads and demands on the mandibular ridge. The clinical consequence of these problems translates to a resorption of the alveolar crest, followed by resorption of the basal bone and finally by an alteration of facial-tissue support. Panoramic radiographs can reveal the amount of remaining bone.

Consultation with a surgeon and restorative dentist is recommended.

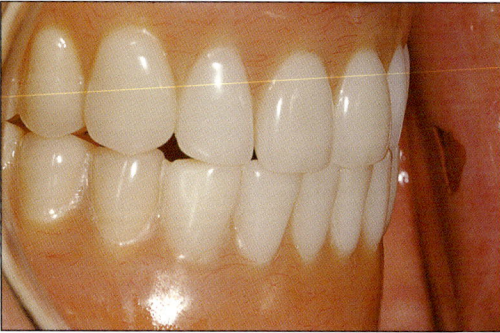

Fig 13-1 A 70-year-old healthy woman has been edentulous since the age of 40 years. She sought treatment because of poor function of her mandibular prosthesis. Her present conventional dentures are 4 years old. In 30 years of wearing conventional dentures, she has never been comfortable with her mandibular denture because it lacks retention and stability, and she has difficulties chewing food. This discomfort has become increasingly apparent in the last 10 years. She is satisfied with the appearance of her maxillary conventional denture and wants to maintain the same tooth arrangement and facial-tissue support.

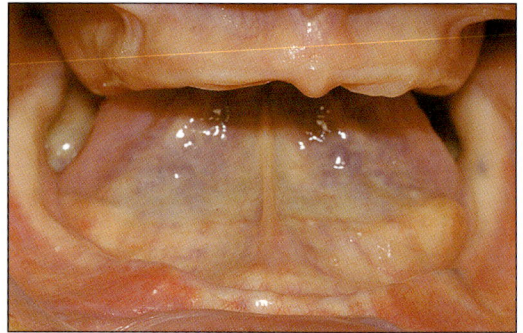

Fig 13-2 Intraoral examination reveals a resorbed and atrophic mandibular ridge that provides minimal denture stability and retention. The midlateral portion of the mandible provides little resistance to dislodgment during denture function. The premolar area is frequently irritated.

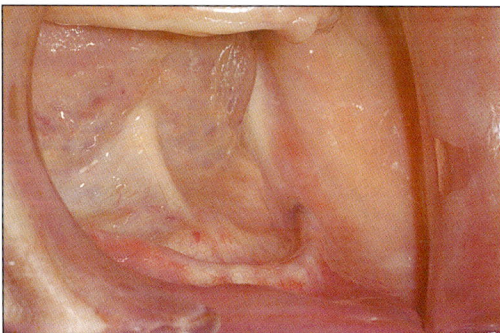

Fig 13-3 The anterior mandibular area has a thin bony ridge. The sagittal interarch relationship is relatively normal but displays a slightly anterior mandible. Interarch space is greater than normal.

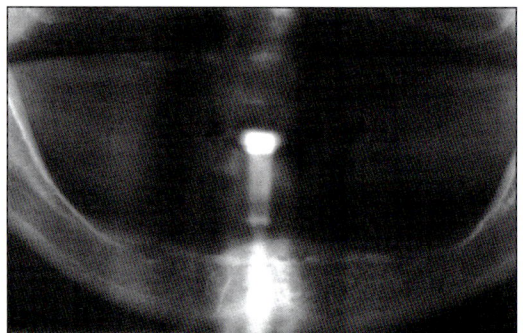

Fig 13-4 The remaining bone corresponds to a type C bone quantity and a type III bone quality.[10] The mental foramina were located on the surface of the ridge, which may contribute to this patient's discomfort during mastication.

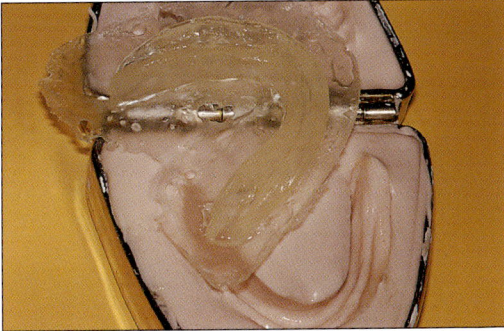

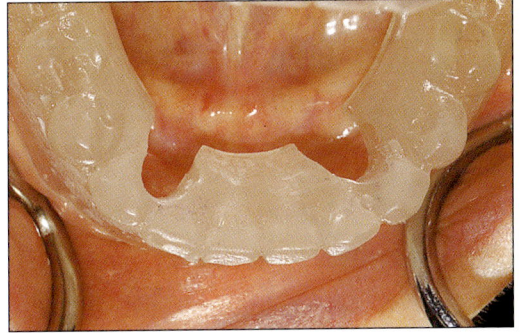

Figs 13-5 and 13-6 A surgical stent is fabricated by duplicating the mandibular denture with orthodontic resin *(left)*. Two vertical grooves are drilled on the lingual surface in the canine areas *(right)*. The anterior position of the implants permits rotation of only the posterior segment of the overdenture. It is important that the rotation axis created by the two implants be parallel to a line through the retromolar pads to allow the overdenture to rotate freely.

Implant Placement

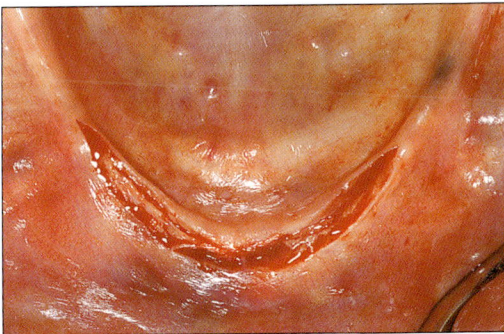

Fig 13-7 A midcrestal incision is made and extended between the first premolar areas. The incision may be limited by the presence of the mental foramina.

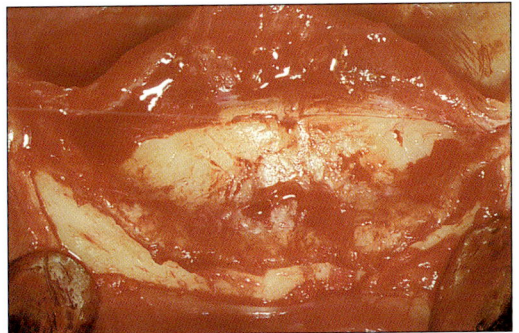

Fig 13-8 Buccal and lingual full-thickness flaps are elevated to expose the residual osseous crest. This surgical approach allows visibility of the ridge morphology and enables the surgeon to modify its shape prior to implant placement.

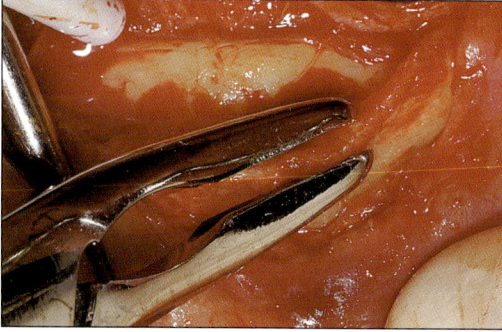

Fig 13-9 The residual osseous crest may need to be eliminated. This provides a more favorable recipient site and minimizes the chance of labial or lingual bony dehiscences.

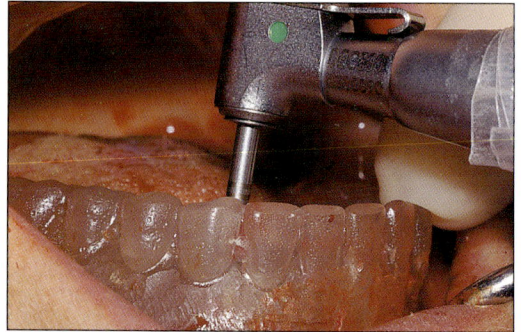

Fig 13-10 The surgical stent allows for appropriate orientation during preparation of the implant site. In this case, both implant sites were prepared for placement of solid screws 10 mm in length.

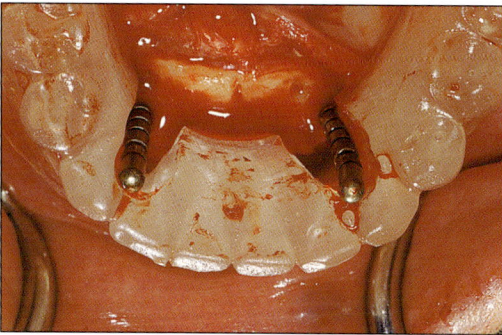

Fig 13-11 Alignment pins (2.2-mm diameter) are inserted into the partially prepared implant sites to verify the orientation relative to the surgical stent.

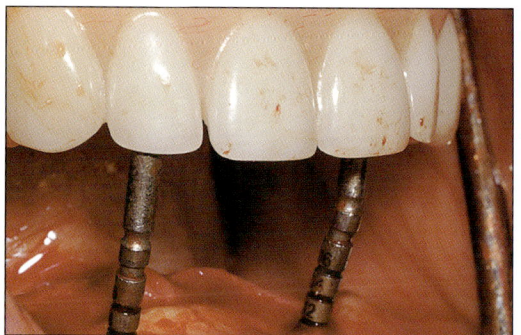

Fig 13-12 Alignment pins also allow the surgeon to evaluate the longitudinal axis of the implants in relation to the incisal edges of the maxillary denture.

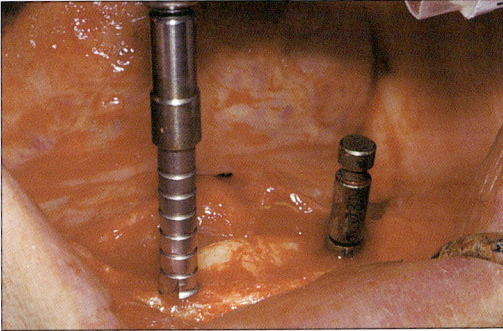

Fig 13-13 The implant sites are then enlarged with a 2.8-mm pilot drill and a 3.5-mm spiral drill, successively. Drilling depth was controlled via clearly visible laser markings on the drilling instruments. The depth can then be verified with a depth gauge. Final site preparation is completed with tapping of the implant site. The screw tap and depth gauges are also marked to allow determination of insertion depth.

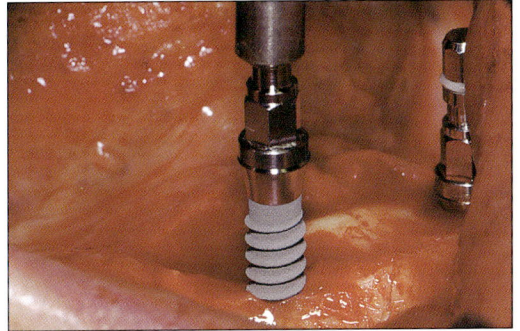

Fig 13-14 Two 4.1 mm x 10 mm solid screw implants with a sandblasted, large-grit, acid-etched (SLA) surface are inserted into their respective sites with a ratchet, under constant irrigation.

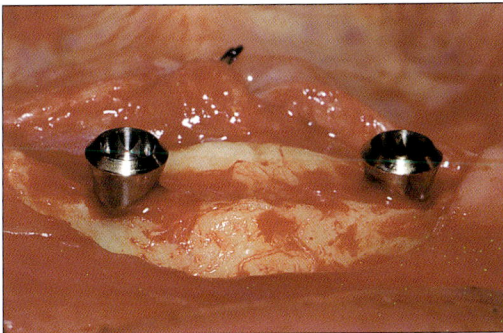

Fig 13-15 For ball-retained mandibular overdentures supported by two implants, implant placement is limited such that the SLA surface is submerged just below the ridge crest.[11] Overseating of the implant in the recipient site should be avoided in order to maximize the length of the transgingival portion of the implant collar.

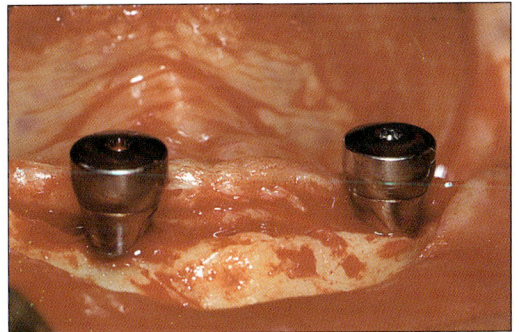

Fig 13-16 Healing caps (4.0-mm diameter) are secured into position. Their height should be sufficient to prevent gingival overgrowth during the healing phase. Healing caps that are too long can interfere with seating of the provisional mandibular denture.

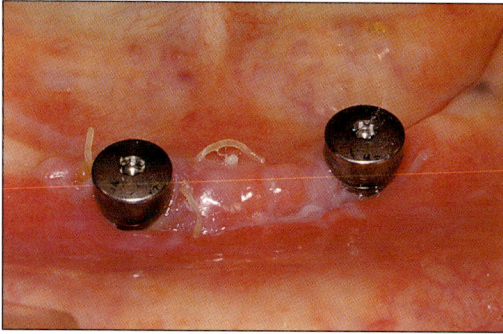

Fig 13-17 Primary closure of the wound is achieved by adaptation of the buccal and lingual flaps around the healing caps.[12] Resorbable or non-resorbable sutures may be used. Ideally, patients should be instructed not to wear the mandibular prosthesis for 2 weeks to avoid disturbing the surgical site during the initial healing phase.

Postsurgical Appointment

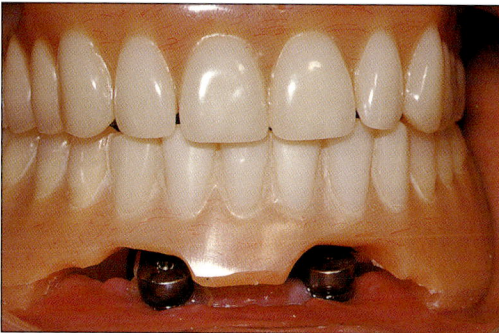

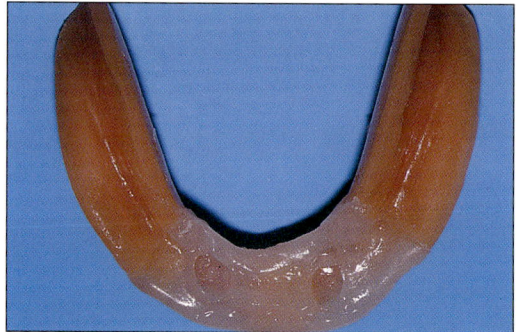

Fig 13-18 Two weeks following implant placement, the anterior portion of the denture is relieved over the healing caps. This procedure allows sufficient space in the denture for a soft relining material (Visco-gel, Dentsply DeTrey, Surrey, United Kingdom) and ensures a healthy relationship between the gingiva and the healing abutments.

Fig 13-19 The patient is dismissed with a functional mandibular denture.

Fig 13-20 After 3 months, the healing abutments are removed, and the ball attachments are torqued into the implants.

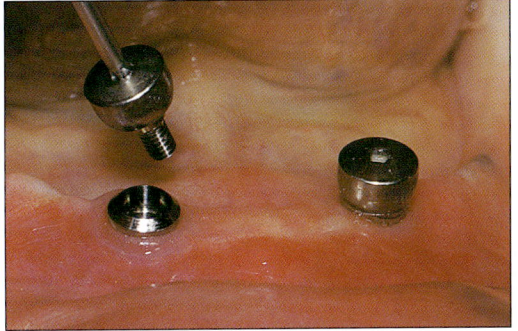

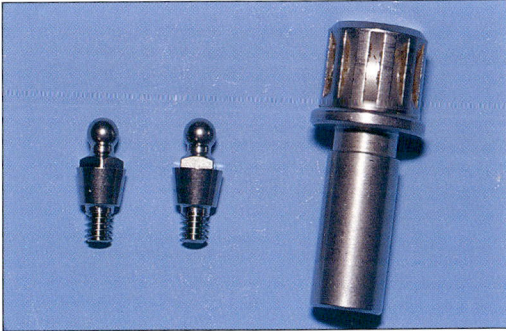

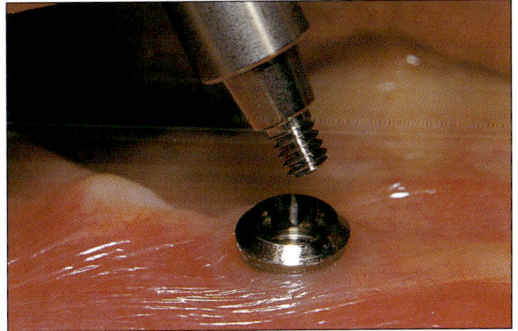

Figs 13-21 and 13-22 The retentive anchor driver is used to secure the abutment into the implants.

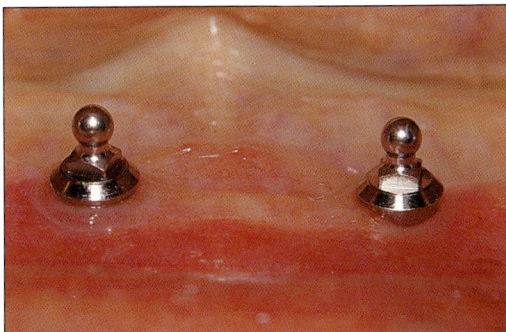

Fig 13-23 Two retentive anchors are joined to the implants.

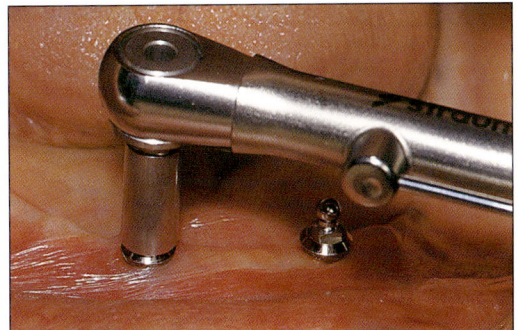

Fig 13-24 A torque driver is used to tighten the ball attachments at 35 N/cm to insure proper seating and resistance to dislodgment.

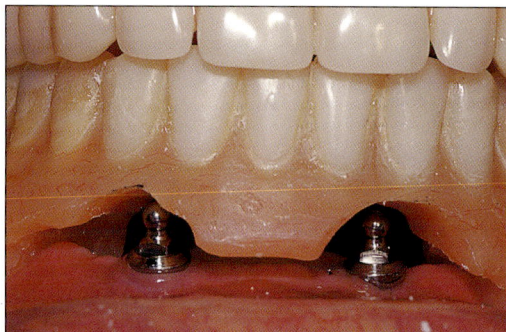

Fig 13-25 The soft tissue reline is grounded off, and the denture base is relieved over the ball attachments.

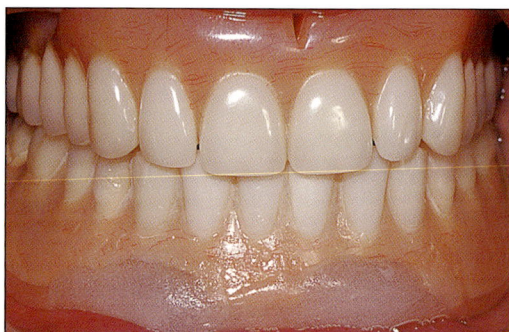

Fig 13-26 New reline material is added to improve denture adaptation and to increase patient comfort.

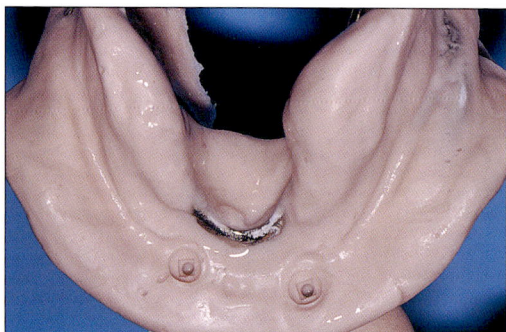

Fig 13-27 Primary alginate impressions of both arches are taken and poured with stone.

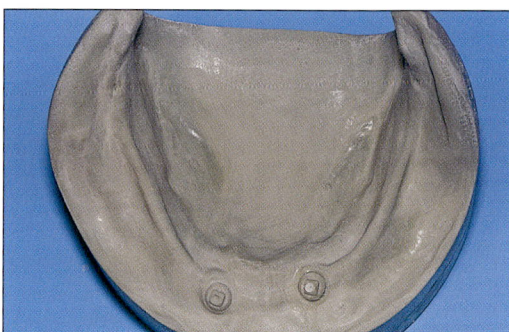

Fig 13-28 The primary casts are used to fabricate custom trays for final impressions.

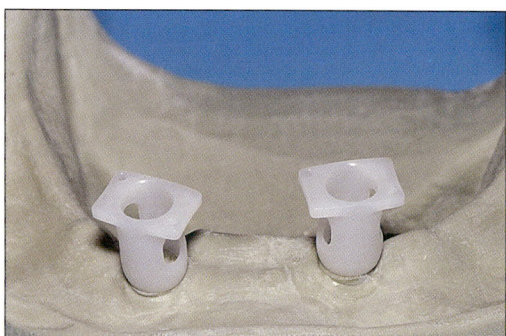

Fig 13-29 Two plastic impression copings are positioned over the ball attachments.

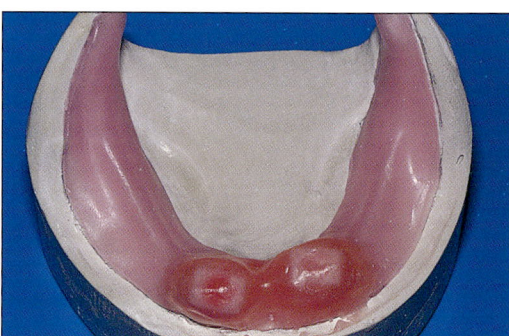

Fig 13-30 A sheet of wax is placed over the ridge and the impression copings to create space in the tray for the impression material.

Fig 13-31 Plastic impression copings are snapped into position over the ball attachments. Special care must be taken to ensure that no calculus or debris interferes with the correct placement of the white plastic copings. The wings of the impression copings may be ground partially and the copings rotated slightly to avoid interference with the impression tray. The custom tray is border molded using a conventional technique.

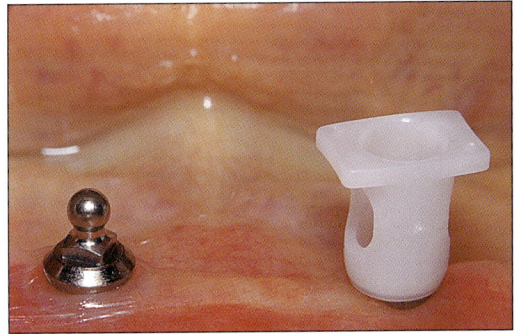

Fig 13-32 A rigid impression material is injected through the coronal orifice of each impression coping, and the impression tray, filled with the same material, is placed in the mouth. Polyether provides rigidity to lock in and pick up the impression copings in their exact position in the mouth.

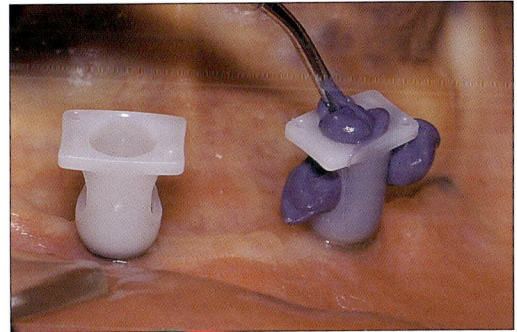

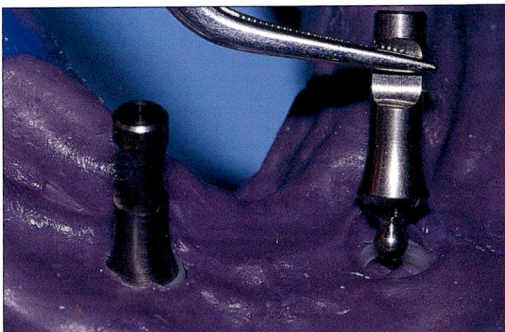

Fig 13-33 Two retentive anchor analogs are snapped in the impression copings.

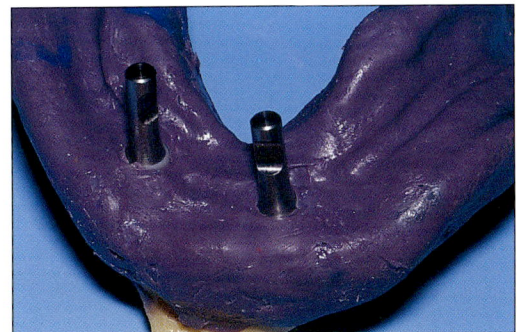

Fig 13-34 If the impression copings are placed correctly on the abutments in the mouth, no impression material should interfere with the placement of the analogs.

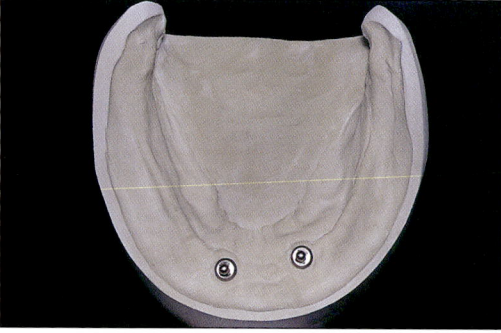

Fig 13-35 The impression is poured with reinforced stone to produce a master cast. A final impression of the maxilla is also taken at this appointment.

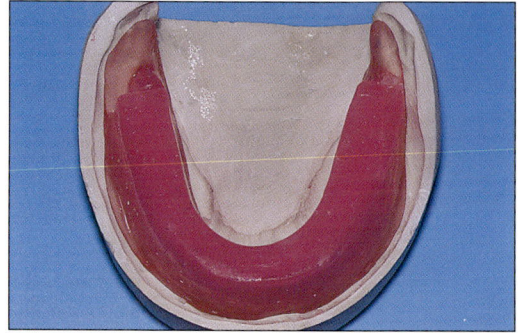

Fig 13-36 Maxillary and mandibular baseplates with wax rims are fabricated for interocclusal registration.

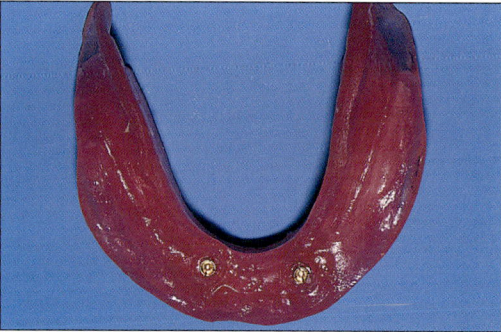

Fig 13-37 Two female matrices, adjusted to minimum retention, are incorporated into the mandibular baseplate to ensure adequate position on the mandibular arch. Simultaneous correct seating of the mandibular baseplate and its matrix–retentive anchor connections is essential to establish a precise occlusal scheme on the dentures.

Third Restorative Appointment

Fig 13-38 The contours and height of the upper wax rim are adjusted. The female matrices of the mandibular baseplate should precisely engage the ball attachments. The contours and height of the mandibular wax rim are adjusted in centric relation at the vertical dimension of the patient. Additional wax is then removed, and two bilateral notches are created on the posterior sextants. An interocclusal record is taken with a bite-registration silicone material in the posterior regions while the patient's mandible is closed in centric relation until an anterior contact is established on the opposing wax rims. Acrylic tooth shape and color are chosen with the patient.

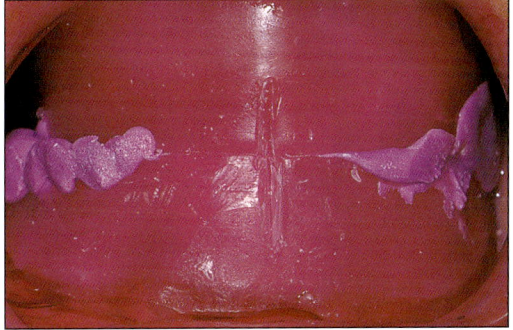

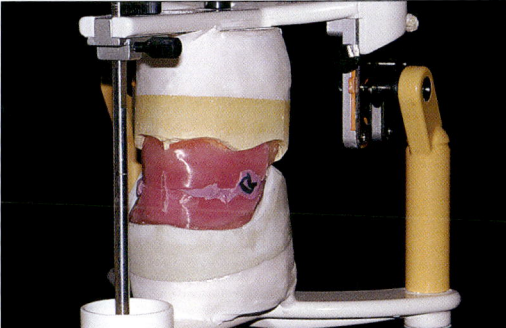

Fig 13-39 The maxillary master cast and baseplate are mounted on a semiadjustable articulator with a facebow. The mandibular cast and baseplate are then mounted on the articulator using the bite-registration index.

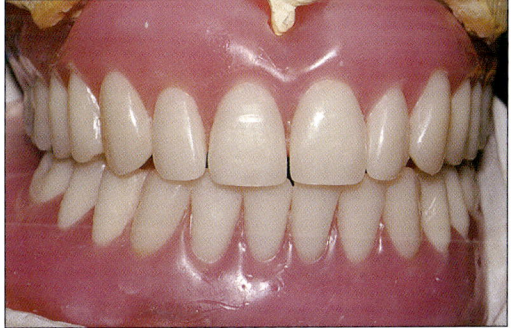

Fig 13-40 Tooth arrangement is similar to the patient's previous dentures. The occlusion follows the fully balanced occlusal concepts and provides better stability of both the maxillary and mandibular dentures in lateral and protrusive excursions.

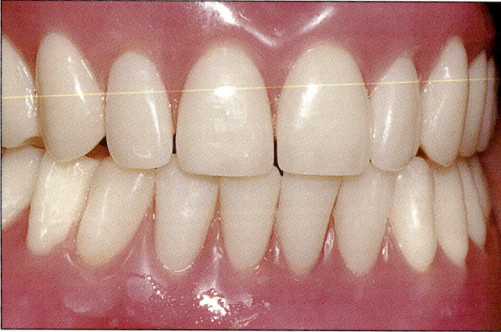

Fig 13-41 The maxillary denture and the mandibular ball-retained overdenture are tried in the mouth. Occlusion, lip and facial support, overdenture tissue adaptation, and ball attachment function are evaluated.

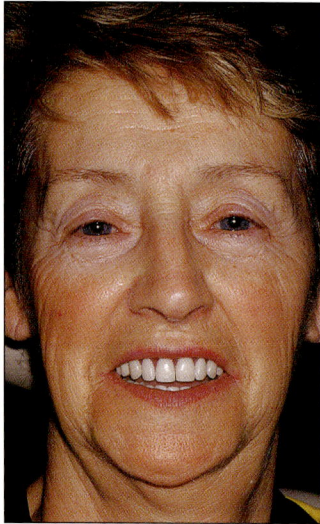

Fig 13-42 If required, tooth arrangement, color, and general esthetics can be modified to meet patient satisfaction and function.

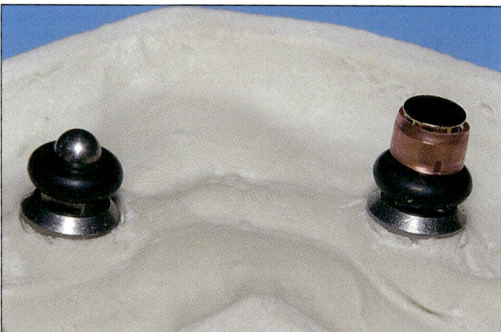

Fig 13-43 The female matrices are recovered from the mandibular baseplate and inserted on the ball attachments. Before the acrylic denture base is processed, a rubber ring is inserted apically onto the female matrix on the analog to prevent denture acrylic from flowing into this area during processing and interfering with the ball attachment mechanism.

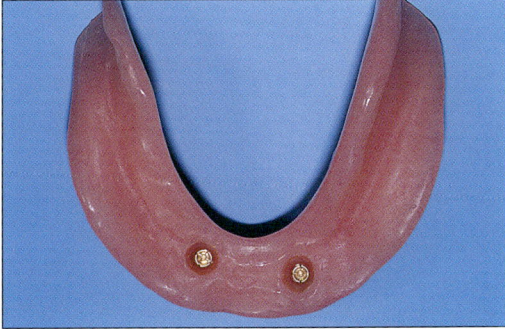

Fig 13-44 The matrices should be adjusted moderately upon denture delivery. Patients need time to become accustomed to insertion and removal of their ball-retained overdentures.

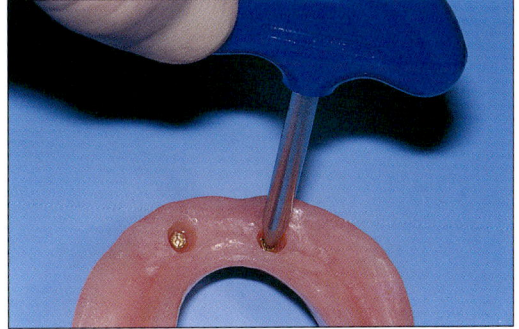

Fig 13-45 If more retention is required, a gold matrix activator is available.

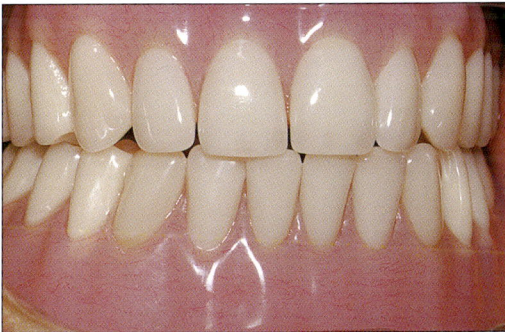

Fig 13-46 The occlusion receives final adjustments in centric relation and during all mandibular movements. A fully balanced concept is adopted to prevent prosthesis instability and dislodgment.

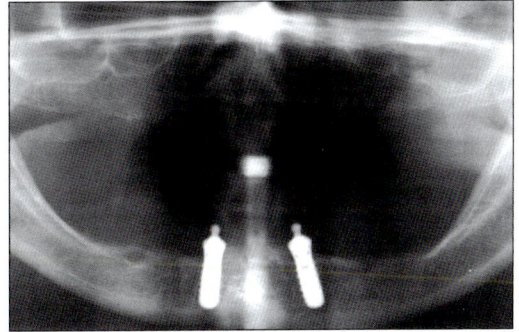

Fig 13-47 This panoramic radiograph illustrates implants and retentive anchors.

Fig 13-48 Patients are instructed to remove their prostheses at night and to clean them properly. Gingival health should be maintained, and the ball attachments should be kept free from calculus and other debris by brushing gently with a soft toothbrush.

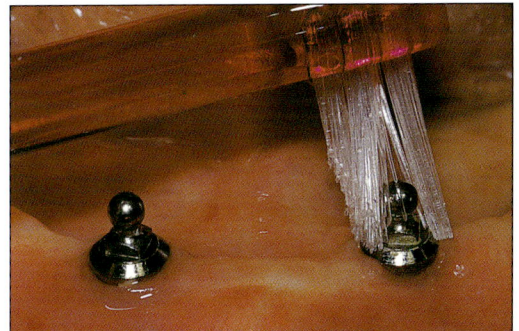

141

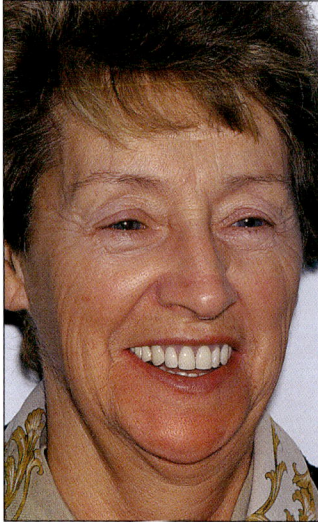

Fig 13-49 The patient is seen for a final control appointment 2 weeks after denture delivery to ensure satisfaction and comfort. Oral hygiene is monitored and reinforced.

Recall Appointments

Recall appointments should be scheduled once every year. Clinical follow-ups should include periapical radiographs of the implants; an evaluation of matrix function and retention; occlusal adjustments, if required; examination of the soft tissues supporting the overdenture and surrounding the attachments; and monitoring of oral hygiene. If calculus deposits are present, a rigid plastic instrument is preferred to enable cleaning without damage to the metal surface.

Summary

Ball-retained overdentures are a favorable treatment option and an affordable implant prosthesis option for patients who are dissatisfied with the retention and stability of their conventional mandibular denture. The following clinical and technical rules should be followed to improve the overdenture function:

1. A thin and narrow residual osseous crest should be eliminated to improve the surgical implant site and to avoid bone dehiscence on the facial and lingual surfaces.
2. The two implants should be located in the canine area. Implants positioned in the premolar areas will displace the rotation axis to the posterior, causing an anterior rotational movement and discomfort to the gingival mucosa.
3. The SLA surface should be submerged slightly below the osseous crest of the ridge to maintain the smooth transgingival por-

tion of the implants in contact with the gingiva and to maximize the position (height) of the retentive anchors (ball attachments) in relation to the gingival level.

4. Before initiating restorative procedures, the retentive anchors must be tightened to 35 N/cm to insure proper seating in the implants.

5. During the impression appointment, care must be taken to correctly place the plastic impression copings on the retentive anchors. Furthermore, to avoid displacement, the coronal wings of these copings should not touch the impression tray. Failure to follow these rules will produce a faulty master cast and an ill-fitting overdenture.

6. The female matrices should be incorporated into the baseplate of the overdenture waxup to verify proper seating and function of the ball attachment mechanism as well as occlusion.

References

1. Mericske-Stern R. Treatment outcomes with implant-supported overdentures: Clinical considerations. J Prosthet Dent 1998;79:66–73.

2. Wismeijer D, van Waas MA, Vermeeren JI, Mulder J, Kalk W. Patient satisfaction with implant-supported mandibular overdentures. A comparison of three treatment strategies with ITI dental implants. Int J Oral Maxillofac Implants 1997;26:263–267.

3. Awad MA, Locker D, Korner-Batinsky N, Feine JS. Measuring the effect of implant rehabilitation on health related quality of life in a randomized controlled clinical trial. J Dent Res 2000;79:1659–1664.

4. Awad MA, Lund JP, Dufresne E, Feine JS. Comparing the efficacy of mandibular implant-retained overdentures and conventional dentures among middle-aged patients: Satisfaction and functional assessment. Int J Prosthodont 2003;16:117–122.

5. Batenburg RHK, Meijer HJA, Raghoebar GM, Vissink A. Treatment concept for mandibular overdentures supported by endosseous implants: A literature review. Int J Oral Maxillofac Implants 1998;13:539–545.

6. Sadowsky SJ. Mandibular implant-retained overdentures: A literature review. J Prosthet Dent 2001;86:468–473.

7. Mericske-Stern R. Three-dimensional force measurements with mandibular overdentures connected to implants by ball-shaped retentive anchors. A clinical study. Int J Oral Maxillofac Implants 1998;13:36–43.

8. Mericske-Stern R, Zarb GA. Overdentures: An alternative implant methodology for edentulous patients. Int J Prosthodont 1993;6:203–208.

9. Mericske-Stern R, Piotti M, Sirtes G. 3-D in vivo force measurements on mandibular implants supporting overdentures. A comparative study. Clin Oral Implants Res 1996;7:387–396.

10. Lekholm U, Zarb GA. Patient selection and preparation. In: Brånemark PI, Zarb GA, Albrektsson T (eds). Tissue-Integrated Prostheses: Osseointegration in Clinical Dentistry. Chicago: Quintessence, 1985:199–209.

11. Buser D, von Arx T, ten Bruggenkate C, Weingart D. Basic surgical principles with ITI implants. Clin Oral Implants Res 2000;11(suppl):59–68.

12. Buser D, Merickse-Stern R, Dual K, Lang NP. Clinical experience with one-stage, nonsubmerged dental implants. Adv Dent Res 1999;13:153–161.

CHAPTER 14

Future Directions

Gunnar E. Carlsson

The development of modern implant dentistry has been extremely rapid. The admirable clinical achievements based on osseointegrated implants have occurred within slightly more than 30 years. It was only 20 years ago that the osseointegration concept was first introduced in North America. The rapid changes of implant dentistry make it difficult to speculate on future directions of implant dentistry.

At a conference in Toronto in 1982, Dr Per-Ingvar Brånemark presented osseointegration and its experimental and clinical background based on more than 2 decades of research and clinical experience.[1] (He placed the first osseointegrated implants in a human patient in 1965!) This started a remarkable worldwide evolution of treatments with osseointegrated implants that has dramatically changed many areas of clinical dentistry and revolutionized prosthodontic therapy for completely and partially edentulous patients. The enormous growth of interest in dental implants is evident in numerous books and journal articles, as well as in a variety of conferences, courses, and symposia. A search in Medline/PubMed in May 2002 listed approximately 6,000 references for "dental implants" and slightly fewer when "prostheses" was added.

During the early period, the Brånemark group considered prosthodontic treatment associated with implants synonymous with fixed implant-supported prostheses. It is well established that this system provides great benefits of oral function and quality of life for edentulous patients with denture problems. However, such treatment is expensive and available only to a small portion of edentulous patients. Less costly alternatives were needed. Therefore, when osseointegrated implants entered the international arena, other prosthodontic alternatives were introduced and tested. Implant-supported or -retained overdentures were described in 1985 in the first textbook on "tissue-integrated implants."[2] In the broadened arsenal of implant-related prosthodontic solutions, implant overdentures have become an important and increasingly common alternative. This treatment modality has been investigated widely during the past few years, and reviews of the growing literature confirm that implant overdentures are a successful prosthetic treatment.[3–5] In May 2002, PubMed revealed 660 references for implant overdentures, demonstrating the rapid growth of this section of implant literature.

The relevant literature has been well reviewed in this book, with a focus on mandibular implant overdentures. The main findings can be summarized as follows:

- Treatment with mandibular implant overdentures, in general, is very successful. However, routine maintenance is required to ensure long-term success.
- Implant survival is high and comparable to that for fixed prostheses.
- Patient satisfaction levels are high.
- The treatment procedure is relatively simple, and the prosthodontic treatment time is similar to that for conventional complete dentures.
- The initial treatment costs are low compared to fixed prostheses.
- Various attachment systems can be used with similar success.

Even if there is near consensus regarding most of the above statements according to the literature reviews, controversy persists concerning treatment concepts and indications for mandibular implant overdentures. Some issues are still debated among clinicians, eg, number of implants, anchorage design, immediate loading, maintenance aspects, patient satisfaction, long-term costs of different retention systems, and removable versus fixed prostheses. Efforts at finding evidenced-based answers to these concerns will be important in the future of implant dentistry. Furthermore, new problems certainly will appear. The solutions will be found in continuing research in close collaboration with clinical activity and development.

Trends and Possible Goals for Mandibular Implant Overdentures

Patient Satisfaction and Masticatory Function

At a conference in Toronto in 1998, a critical review of literature on the patient-based outcomes of implant therapy surprised the audience. What every prosthodontist considered evident—the great benefits of implant-supported prostheses—was questioned because most studies had design flaws that threatened their internal validity.[6] The reviewer noted that, from a strictly scientific point of view, the studies conducted up to 1998 provided relatively little scientific evidence that implant therapy is of substantially more benefit to edentulous patients than alternative forms of treatment. It was concluded that further research was needed using randomized controlled trial (RCT) designs. Outcome measures need to be more carefully selected so as to reflect patients' concerns. More recent studies have addressed patient satisfaction and verified that patients with implant overdentures had higher satisfaction scores than complete denture wearers, even in comparison with those who had preprosthetic surgery to enlarge the denture-bearing area.[7] In one of the recent studies using patient-based assessments (eg, Oral Health Impact Profile, or OHIP), it was found that patients who chose complete dentures when implant overdentures also were available reported significant improvement after treatment, as did those who received implant treatment. Both groups reported much greater improvement compared to the patients who requested implants but received complete dentures.[8] During the past few years, a series of

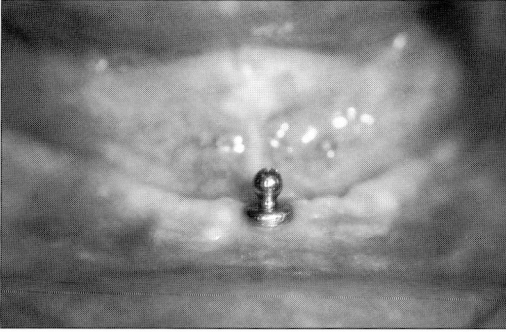

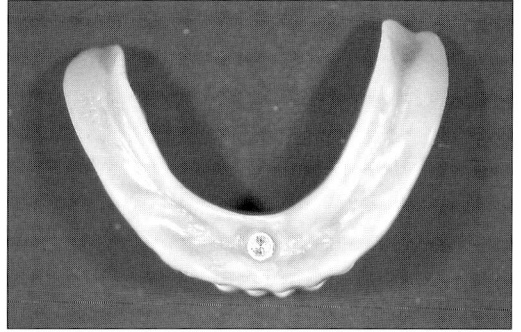

Figs 14-1a and 14-1b Single midline implant to retain a mandibular overdenture. (Reprinted from Krennmair and Ulm[16] with permission.)

RCTs have shown higher satisfaction and oral health–related quality of life among patients with implant overdentures than among those with conventional dentures (see chapter 5).

Cross-over studies have been conducted for comparison of fixed versus removable implant-supported prostheses. The removable design was selected (by half of the patients) for ease of cleaning, among other reasons, whereas the fixed prosthesis was chosen because it provided better stability and ability to chew.[9] There was no difference in general satisfaction between the fixed and removable treatments, but patients found the fixed prosthesis to be better for chewing harder foods.[10] Improvements in bite force and chewing efficiency following implant treatment in edentulous patients has been demonstrated for many years,[11] and similar results for mandibular implant overdentures have been presented.[12]

Number of Implants

The theory that more implants will better support a heavy functional load may be true from a theoretical biomechanical point of view, and it explains the early uncertainty about how many implants to use for supporting or retaining an overdenture. However, numerous clinical prospective studies up to 12 years have proven that two mandibular intraforaminal implants, splinted or unsplinted, retaining an overdenture provide successful treatment for edentulous mandibles.[5,13,14]

A few studies have compared mandibular overdentures supported by two, three, or four implants. Results indicate that two implants are sufficient, in general, and this seems to be the most common choice today. The recommendations to use more than two implants in special situations[5] appear to be based on speculation rather than on results of controlled clinical studies. Such studies would be desirable to provide a better basis for decision making. However, there is consensus that, for the great majority of edentulous patients, two intraforaminal implants are sufficient for a successful mandibular implant overdenture.

The possibility of reducing the number of implants to one has been tested in a 5-year prospective study of 21 elderly patients.[15] None of the implants was lost during the follow-up period and "remarkable improvement of oral comfort and function was evidenced with the overdenture treatment." Similar success was reported in a more recent investigation with fewer patients and a shorter observation period (Figs 14-1a and 14-1b).[16] The

Table 14-1 Comparison of the most common retention systems for mandibular implant overdentures according to current literature

Variable	Bar-clip	Ball
Implant survival	+	+
Peri-implant bone loss	+	+
Retention	+	–
Hygiene	–	+
Cost/simplicity	?	?
Maintenance	?	?
Patient satisfaction	+	+

(+) Advantage; (–) disadvantage; (?) inconclusive results.

authors of both studies emphasized the benefit of their method, especially for geriatric patients with severe denture problems, because it is relatively inexpensive and is a surgically and prosthodontically simple way of retaining a complete denture. In spite of these successful results, the method with only one implant does not seem to have become more widely accepted. However, this alternative deserves to be investigated using an RCT that compares the outcome of complete dentures to mandibular overdentures anchored to one implant.

Retention Systems

Several retention systems for implant overdentures have been described in the literature. However, for mandibular overdentures supported by two implants, the implants can be interconnected with a bar or remain unsplinted. The first implant overdentures used a bar-clip attachment, but the use of unsplinted implants has increased. Currently, unsplinted implants with ball attachments are the most common system, but the choice of a specific system can

be based more on subjective preferences than scientific evidence. In vitro studies have reported conflicting results regarding stresses and loading on implants and surrounding bone with different splinted and unsplinted retention systems. However, several clinical longitudinal studies have found no differences in implant survival and peri-implant variables.[17–19]

If implant survival rates do not differ among the retention systems, other factors may be important. Implant overdentures have been shown to require substantial prosthodontic maintenance, especially during the first year of service. Whether the splinted or unsplinted design requires more maintenance is controversial, and the literature is not conclusive regarding comparisons between bar-clip and ball attachments (Table 14-1). Magnets on unsplinted implants also have been used to retain overdentures, but the retention is poorer, which can influence patient satisfaction.[13] A recent study demonstrated that ball attachments of three different implant systems required different amounts of maintenance, even if the overall prosthetic maintenance was similar. Two out of three patients required prosthetic maintenance in the first year and the matrices of two of the studied implant systems "showed problems of clinical significance."[20] Time and cost implications should be included in the economic aspects of the various treatments. One study estimated the cost for prosthetic and laboratory service at US $218 per patient over a 3-year period.[21]

Immediate Loading

The extremely successful results with osseointegrated implants placed according to the two-stage procedure have led to attempts to reduce healing time. Several studies have demonstrated immediate loading as a successful option for fixed prostheses. The optimal solution is probably the Brånemark Novum technique, which allows patients to receive a mandibular fixed prosthesis supported on three implants on the day of implant surgery.[22] Mandibular implant overdentures loaded immediately or after a short healing time have shown high success rates in a few short-term studies indicating that this may be a promising treatment option (see chapter 12).

Bone Preservation

Complete denture wearers inevitably exhibit continuing bone resorption of the residual ridges.[23] This can be substantially reduced if a fixed implant-supported prosthesis is placed, and several studies claim that such treatment helps preserve the existing residual bony ridge. For patients with implant overdentures, the anterior bone adjacent to the implants resorbs very little; there are conflicting reports regarding the effect on the posterior residual ridge. A recent study concluded that patients rehabilitated with mandibular fixed prostheses demonstrated bone apposition in the poste-

rior mandibular region, whereas those with implant overdentures showed low rates of residual ridge resorption.[24] Bone resorption does not appear to be a serious concern when mandibular implant overdentures are used, but the restoration of some of the previously resorbed bone, as seen with fixed implant-supported prostheses, is an exciting possibility.

Epidemiology and Demographics

The rate of edentulism is rapidly declining in most countries. An example of the ongoing dramatic change occurring in Sweden is demonstrated in Fig 14-2.[25] This decline usually has been interpreted so that the number of edentulous people will decrease. However, recent analyses combining epidemiologic and demographic data indicate that the number of people in the United States who need complete dentures will actually increase over the next 20 years, despite an anticipated decline in rates of edentulism of approximately 10% per decade.[26] Surprisingly, this article did not discuss the possibility of using implant overdentures or other implant-anchored prostheses. The unexpected growth in the number of edentulous people can be explained by other global trends: the growth of the elderly population and longer life expectancy. Figure 14-3 demonstrates the changes of the age pyramid of Sweden over 135 years, but the situation is similar in many countries (see chapter 1).

Under these conditions, the market for implant overdentures appears promising. It must be remembered, however, that until recently, implant therapy has been limited to a small portion of the population. In 1997, it was estimated that 2 million people had received some form of implant treatment, which corresponds to less than 1 person per 1,000 of the global population with tooth loss.[23] A report from the dental implant industry in April 2002

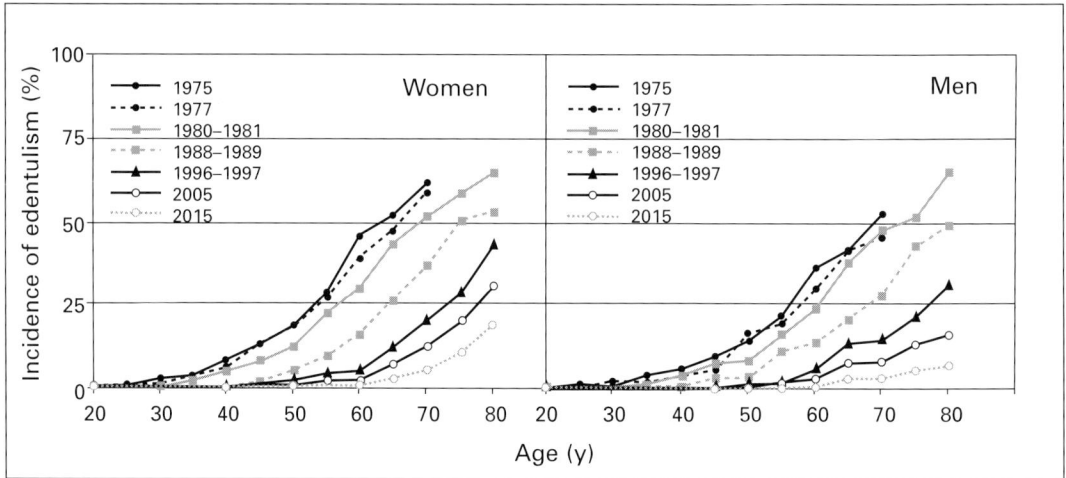

Fig 14-2 Changes in edentulism in Swedish women and men from 1975 to 1997 and with prognosis up to 2015. (Modified from Österberg[25] with permission from Taylor & Francis.)

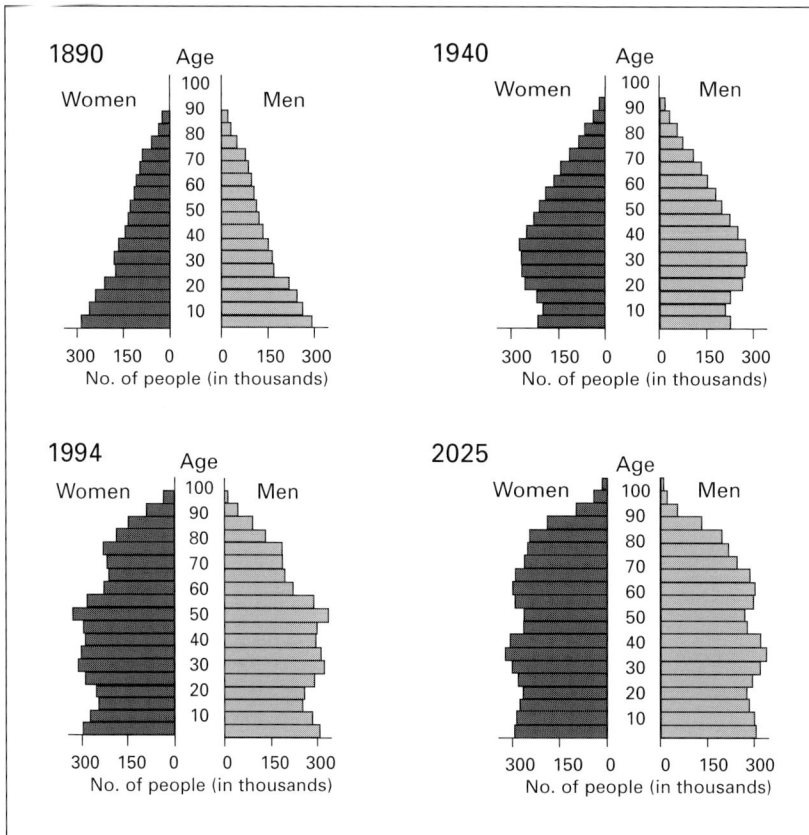

Fig 14-3 Changes of the age pyramid for Sweden over 135 years.

Table 14-2 Comparison of implant overdentures (IOD) and complete dentures (CD) according to current literature

Variable	IOD	CD
Patient satisfaction	+	–
Bite force	+	–
Chewing efficiency	+	–
Initial cost	–	+
Maintenance cost	–	+

(+) Advantage; (–) disadvantage.

estimated that about 3 million people through the year 2001 had been treated with dental implants, corresponding to only 3% of edentulous people in the United States (Chattwal A, et al, unpublished data, 2002). This report calculated the annual increase of the implant market at 13% to 15%, but there is very little documentation in the literature of implant epidemiology. No available data repudiate the fact that, over the next few decades, the great majority of completely and partially edentulous patients will continue to receive conventional prosthodontic treatments. It remains a heavy task for those who wish to promote wider use of implant-supported overdentures or other implant-supported restorations.

Implant Overdentures Versus Fixed Implant Prostheses

The literature provides strong evidence that an implant overdenture is a very successful treatment alternative for the edentulous mandible in comparison with complete dentures (Table 14-2). Cost is the only factor that makes complete dentures more favorable. Even if the use of implant overdentures is growing rapidly, the concept is not yet universally accepted. In Sweden, for example, implant overdenture treatment is rare and fixed prostheses still are the most common implant therapy for edentulous mandibles. A survey of specialized prosthodontic clinics in Sweden found that several clinics did not perform this treatment at all, and the median number of overdentures provided per clinic in 2001 was 2, whereas the corresponding figure for fixed implant prostheses was 17.[27] One explanation is perhaps the preference for fixed rather than removable prostheses, which may be partly related to a favorable Swedish dental insurance system. The interpretation of available results regarding advantages and disadvantages of fixed and removable implant restorations (Table 14-3) may vary depending on, for example, economic and cultural background factors.

Determination of future directions for treatment of mandibular edentulism requires a comparison of the main alternatives. The traditional complete denture has been a fairly successful treatment for a majority of edentulous patients and most likely will continue into the foreseeable future in a global perspective. With respect to demographic changes such as the growth of the elderly population, which leads to an increased number of edentulous patients, conventional complete denture treat-

Table 14-3 Comparison of implant overdentures (IOD) to fixed implant-supported prostheses (FISP) according to current literature

Variable	IOD	FISP
Patient satisfaction	+	+
Bite force	–	+
Chewing efficiency	–	+
Initial cost	+	–
Maintenance cost	?	?

(+) Advantage; (–) disadvantage; (?) inconclusive results.

Table 14-4 Comparison of mandibular implant overdentures (IOD), fixed implant-supported prostheses (FISP), and complete dentures (CD)

Variable	IOD	FISP	CD
Treatment simplicity/availability	+	–	++
Initial treatment cost	+	–	++
Maintenance cost (first year)	?	?	+
Maintenance cost long-term	?	?	+
Long-term treatment success (over 10 years)	+	++	–
Long-term implant survival	+	++	NA
Hygienic aspects	+	–	++
Masticatory function (bite force, chewing efficiency)	+	++	–
Patient preference	+	++	+
Bone preservation	+	++	–
Immediate loading	?	+	NA
Dentist factors	+	++	–
Patient factors	++	++	+

(++, +) Advantages; (–) disadvantage; (?) inconclusive results; (NA) not applicable.

ment continues to be important despite the decreasing rate of edentulism (see chapter 1). The proven possibility of implants to overcome several shortcomings of complete dentures will most probably result in a continuing increase of implant-anchored prostheses. The international distribution of removable and fixed implant prostheses is not well known and more epidemiologic data are needed. The literature reveals that the use of implant overdentures is increasing in many countries, whereas fixed implant prostheses are preferred in others.

A comparison of the three alternatives for treatment of mandibular edentulism is presented in Table 14-4. Even if the advantages are based on available literature, interpretation is subjective. A simple tabulation of the "+" marks does not indicate which alternative is the best. Individual arguments and evaluations should be included in decision making. However, the table may explain part of the complexity of the decision process. It may also indicate why complete dentures still are a realistic, and necessary, alternative for many edentulous patients. The relatively positive reaction to complete dentures among edentulous patients, demonstrated in many studies,[23] may be due in part to "satisfaction on a too low level." Many complete denture wearers might reach a higher level of satisfaction—and quality of life—if they could try implant overdentures. It is an important task for the dental profession to inform edentulous patients of the implant overdenture alternative and to make it more readily available and affordable to this growing population.

Summary

It has been suggested that implant overdentures are likely to replace conventional dentures as the preferred mode of prosthetic rehabilitation for edentulous patients. This is an attractive future direction, but will it be realized? Current trends in many countries suggest a relatively good prognosis for such a goal, but there are alternative roads to walk. The enormous development in implant overdenture therapy during the past 20 years will certainly continue, but its direction is not evident. The choice between different treatment options should be evidence based, which requires controlled clinical research, preferably by means of randomized controlled trials. Some topics of interest for such research in the near future include:

- Epidemiologic surveys on edentulism in relation to demographic changes and need and demand for implant treatment
- Long-term randomized controlled trials comparing mandibular implant overdentures and fixed implant prostheses (eg, cost, success rates, patient preference, and patient quality of life)
- Randomized controlled trials comparing complete dentures with mandibular overdentures supported by one and two implants
- Continuing in vitro and in vivo research on implant components to improve the survival and success rate of implant treatment and to reduce maintenance costs

The results of such research will facilitate clinicians' decision making for edentulous patients and will help them reach the ultimate goal of improving the quality of life for these edentulous patients.

References

1. Brånemark PI. Osseointegration and its experimental background. J Prosthet Dent 1983;50:399–410.
2. Brånemark PI, Zarb GA, Albrektsson T. Tissue-Integrated Prostheses. Chicago: Quintessence,1985.
3. Batenburg RH, Meijer HJ, Raghoebar GM, Vissink A. Treatment concept for mandibular overdentures supported by endosseous implants: A literature review. Int J Oral Maxillofac Implants 1998;13:539–545.
4. Payne AGT, Solomons YF. The prosthodontic maintenance requirements of the mandibular mucosa- and implant-supported overdentures: A review of literature. Int J Prosthodont 2000;13:238–245.

5. Sadowsky SJ. Mandibular implant-retained overdentures: A literature review. J Prosthet Dent 2001; 86:468–473.

6. Locker D. Patient-based assessment of the outcomes of implant therapy: A review of the literature. Int J Prosthodont 1998;11:453–461.

7. Raghoebar GM, Meijer HJ, Stegenga B, van't Hof MA, van Oort RP, Vissink A. Effectiveness of three treatment modalities for the edentulous mandible. A five-year randomized clinical trial. Clin Oral Implants Res 2000;11:195–201.

8. Allen PF, McMillan AS, Walshaw D. A patient-based assessment of implant-stabilized and conventional complete dentures. J Prosthet Dent 2001;85: 141–147.

9. Feine JS, de Grandmont P, Boudrias P, et al. Within-subject comparisons of implant-supported mandibular prostheses: Choice of prosthesis. J Dent Res 1994;73:1105–1111.

10. de Grandmont P, Feine JS, Tache R, et al. Within-subject comparisons of implant-supported mandibular prostheses: Psychometric evaluation. J Dent Res 1994;73:1096–1104.

11. Haraldson T, Carlsson GE. Bite force and oral function in patients with osseointegrated oral implants. Scand J Dent Res 1977;85:200–208.

12. van Kampen FM, van der Bilt A, Cune MS, Bosman F. The influence of various attachment types in mandibular implant-retained overdentures on maximum bite force and EMG. J Dent Res 2002;81: 170–173.

13. Davis DM, Packer ME. Mandibular overdentures stabilized by Astra Tech implants with either ball or magnets: 5-year results. Int J Prosthodont 1999;12: 222–229.

14. van Steenberghe D, Quirynen M, Naert I, Maffei G, Jacobs R. Marginal bone loss around implants retaining hinging mandibular overdentures, at 4-, 8- and 12-years follow-up. J Clin Periodontol 2001; 28:628–633.

15. Cordioli G, Najsaub Z, Castagna S. Mandibular overdentures anchored to single implants: A 5-year prospective study. J Prosthet Dent 1997;78:159–165.

16. Krennmair G, Ulm C. The symphyseal single-tooth implant for anchorage of a mandibular complete denture in geriatric patients: A clinical report. Int J Oral Maxillofac Implants 2001;16:98–104.

17. Bergendal T, Engquist B. Implant-supported overdentures: A longitudinal prospective study. Int J Oral Maxillofac Implants 1998;13:253–262.

18. Naert I, Gizani S, Vuylsteke M, van Steenberghe D. A 5-year randomized clinical trial on the influence of splinted and unsplinted oral implants in the mandibular overdenture therapy. Part I: Peri-implant outcome. Clin Oral Implants Res 1998;9:170–177.

19. Gotfredsen K, Holm B. Implant-supported mandibular overdentures retained with ball or bar attachments: A randomized prospective 5-year study. Int J Prosthodont 2000;13:125–130.

20. Watson GK, Payne AGT, Purton DG, Thomson WM. Mandibular overdentures: Comparative evaluation of prosthodontic maintenance of three different implant systems during the first year of service. Int J Prosthodont 2002;15:259–266.

21. Chaffee NR, Felton DA, Cooper LF, Palmqvist U, Smith R. Prosthetic complications in an implant-retained mandibular overdenture population: Initial analysis of a prospective study. J Prosthet Dent 2002;87:40–44.

22. Engstrand P, Nannmark U, Mårtensson L, Galéus I, Brånemark P-I. Brånemark Novum: Prosthodontic and laboratory procedures for fabrication of a fixed prosthesis on the day of surgery. Int J Prosthodont 2001;14:303–309.

23. Carlsson GE. Clinical morbidity and sequelae of treatment with complete dentures. J Prosthet Dent 1998;79:17–23.

24. Wright PS, Glantz PO, Randow K, Watson RM. The effects of fixed and removable implant-stabilised prostheses on posterior mandibular residual ridge resorption. Clin Oral Implants Res 2002;13: 169–174.

25. Österberg T, Carlsson GE, Sundh V. Trends and prognoses of dental status in the Swedish population: Analysis based on interviews in 1975 to 1997 by Statistics Sweden. Acta Odontol Scand 2000;58: 177–182.

26. Douglas CW, Shih A, Ostry L. Will there be a need for complete dentures in the United States in 2020? J Prosthet Dent 2002;87:5–8.

27. Kronström M, Carlsson GE. Use of implant overdentures in edentulous mandibles. A survey of treatment policy in prosthodontic specialist clinics in Sweden. Swed Dent J 2003 (in press).

The McGill Consensus Statement on Overdentures

On May 24–25, 2002, a symposium was held at McGill University in Montreal, Quebec, Canada, during which scientists and expert clinicians presented 15 papers on the efficacy of overdentures for the treatment of edentulous patients. Strong emphasis was given to evidence from randomized controlled trials in which mandibular two-implant overdentures were compared to conventional dentures.

A draft consensus statement was circulated to all presenters, as well as to subjects who participated in some of the clinical trials and to other edentulous individuals who attended the symposium. The statement was modified during the meeting in light of the presenters' comments.

We hope that the final version of the consensus statement will serve as a guideline for clinicians and patients, and that it will stimulate discussion within and between professional organizations, health authorities, and third-party payers.

Mandibular Two-Implant Overdentures as First-Choice Standard of Care for Edentulous Patients

A panel of experts who work in areas relevant to the consensus question, as well as patients and clinical-trial participants who have experience with dental prostheses, prepared this consensus statement. It is based on (1) presentations given by these experts during a 1.5-day session; (2) available scientific knowledge on this topic; and (3) personal experience of the patients and participants. This statement is an independent report and is not a policy statement for any profit-making body or business.

Most industrialized countries are experiencing a rapid decline in tooth loss. However, tooth loss increases with age, so the number of edentulous people within these societies will continue to increase for several decades because of the increase in mean age. Complete maxillary and mandibular dentures have been the traditional standard of care for edentulous patients for more than a century. Complete-denture wearers are usually able to wear a maxillary denture without problems, but many struggle to eat with the complete mandibular denture because it is too mobile. Scientific studies have been carried out over the past decade to determine if the benefit of a mandibular two-implant overdenture is significant enough to propose it, rather than the conventional denture, as the first treatment option.

It has already been established through longitudinal clinical studies, structured reviews, and consensus conferences, that the survival of root-form titanium implants is very high in the anterior mandible and that the incidence of surgical complications is very low. Furthermore, it has been shown that implants reduce the rate of resorption of the residual ridge in the anterior mandible.

Patient Perspective

Conventional dentures rely on the residual alveolar ridge and mucosa for support and retention. Many patients have problems adapting to their complete dentures, especially to the mandibular prosthesis. The widespread use of denture adhesives is one indication that these prostheses are inadequate for many denture wearers. Numerous people wearing conventional dentures report that they cannot eat many foods, particularly those that are hard or tough. This forces them to change their diets in unhealthy ways and causes their nutrition to be poorer than that of people with natural teeth.

Mandibular two-implant overdentures have been shown to be superior to conventional dentures in randomized and nonrandomized clinical trials that ranged in duration from 6 months to 9 years. Regardless of the type of attachment system used (bar, ball, or magnet), participants are significantly more satisfied with two-implant overdentures than with new conventional dentures. Patients find the implant overdentures significantly more stable, and they rate their ability to chew various foods as significantly easier. In addition, they are more comfortable and speak more easily with implant overdentures.

Studies of several populations have shown that ratings of quality of life are significantly higher for patients who receive two-implant overdentures (opposing complete maxillary conventional dentures) than for those with new conventional dentures.

There is emerging evidence that people who receive mandibular two-implant overdentures modify their diets, while those who wear new conventional dentures do not. There is also preliminary evidence that this improves their nutritional state. Such improvements may have a strong positive impact on general health, particularly for senior adults who are vulnerable to malnutrition.

Cost

Moreover, there is now conclusive evidence that oral implants may be placed in a single-stage procedure, which reduces cost. Nevertheless, the total cost of providing mandibular two-implant overdentures is certainly greater than that of conventional dentures. However, the difference is not as large as one might expect and should be made affordable to everyone who is edentate.

Conclusions

The evidence currently available suggests that the restoration of the edentulous mandible with a conventional denture is no longer the most appropriate first-choice prosthodontic treatment. There is now overwhelming evidence that a two-implant overdenture should become the first choice of treatment for the edentulous mandible.

J. S. Feine, DDS, MSc, HDR; Canada

G. E. Carlsson, LDS, Odont Dr (PhD), Dr Odont hc, FDSRCS (Eng); Sweden

M. A. Awad, BDS, MSc, PhD; United Arab Emirates

A. Chehade, BSc, DDS, MSc, FRCD(C); Canada

W. J. Duncan, MDS, FRACDS; New Zealand

S. Gizani, DDS, MDS; Greece

T. Head, DDS, MSc, FRCD(C); Canada

G. Heydecke, DDS, Dr Med Dent; Germany

J. P. Lund, BDS, PhD, Dr Odont hc; Canada

M. MacEntee, LDS(I), FRCD(C), PhD; Canada

R. Mericske-Stern, Dr Med Dent, PhD; Switzerland

P. Mojon, DMD, PhD; Canada

J. A. Morais, MD, FRCPC; Canada

I. Naert, Dr Dent, PhD; Belgium

A. G. T. Payne, BDS, MDent, FCD(SA); New Zealand

J. Penrod, MA, PhD; Canada

G. T. Stoker, Jr, DDS; The Netherlands

Y. Takanashi, DDS, PhD; Japan

A. Tawse-Smith, DDS; New Zealand

T. D. Taylor, DDS, MSD, FACP; United States

J. M. Thomason, BDS, PhD, FDSRCS(Ed); United Kingdom

W. M. Thomson, BSc, BDS, MComDent, MA, PhD; New Zealand

D. Wismeijer, DDS, PhD; The Netherlands

This statement is supported by published studies, which form the basis of the material presented in this book.

Index